THE DIET COOKBOOK (2 BOOKS IN 1)

The complete guide to manage kidney disease and to start an anti-inflammatory diet improving your health with 200+ recipes

Lewis W. Martin

Copyright © 2019 by LEWIS W. MARTIN
All rights reserved.

This document is geared towards providing exact and reliable information with regard to the topic and issue covered. The publication is sold with the idea that the publisher is not required to render accounting, officially permitted, or otherwise, qualified services. If advice is necessary, legal or professional, a practiced individual in the profession should be ordered.

From a Declaration of Principles which was accepted and approved equally by a Committee of the American Bar Association and a Committee of Publishers and Associations.

In no way is it legal to reproduce, duplicate, or transmit any part of this document in either electronic means or in printed format. Recording of this publication is strictly prohibited and any storage of this document is not allowed unless with written permission from the publisher. All rights reserved.

The information provided herein is stated to be truthful and consistent, in that any liability, in terms of inattention or otherwise, by any usage or abuse of any policies, processes, or directions contained within is the solitary and utter responsibility of the recipient reader. Under no circumstances will any legal responsibility or blame be held against the publisher for any reparation, damages, or monetary loss due to the information herein, either directly or indirectly.

Respective authors own all copyrights not held by the publisher.

The information herein is offered for informational purposes solely and is universal as so. The presentation of the information is without a contract or any type of guarantee assurance.

The trademarks that are used are without any consent, and the publication of the trademark is without permission or backing by the trademark owner. All trademarks and brands within this book are for clarifying purposes only and are owned by the owners themselves, not affiliated with this document.

Disclaimer

The content of this book is for informational purposes only and is not intended to diagnose, treat, cure, or prevent any condition or disease. You understand that this book is not intended as a substitute for consultation with a licensed practitioner. Please consult with your own physician or healthcare specialist regarding the suggestions and recommendations made in this book. The use of this book implies your acceptance of this disclaimer.

TABLE OF CONTENTS

STOPPING KIDNEY DISEASE

THE STRUCTURE OF THE KIDNEY 5
CHRONIC KIDNEY WEAKNESS: FIRST SIGNS & SYMPTOMS 14
CHRONIC RENAL INSUFFICIENCY: TREATMENT 22
DIETARY GUIDELINES 34
TOP 15 KIDNEY-FRIENDLY NUTRITION FOR PEOPLE WITH
KIDNEY PROBLEMS 41
STOP SMOKING: 10 PITFALLS AND TIPS. 54
90+ RECIPES 57

ANTI-INFLAMMATORY DIET FOR BEGINNERS

CHAPTER 1: THE ORIGINS OF THE ANTI-INFLAMMATORY
DIET 130
CHAPTER 2: WHAT IS INFLAMMATION AND WHAT CAUSES
IT? 133
CHAPTER 3: LISTS OF ANTI-INFLAMMATORY FOODS 137
CHAPTER 4: WHAT IS AN ANTI-INFLAMMATORY DIET? 144
CHAPTER 5: ANTI-INFLAMMATORY FOODS AND THEIR
HEALTH BENEFITS 146
CHAPTER 6: SIMPLE TECHNIQUES TO FIGHT
INFLAMMATION 149
CHAPTER 7: LISTS OF ANTI-INFLAMMATORY RECIPES 151
CHAPTER 8: BREAKFAST RECIPES 180
CHAPTER 9: SEAFOOD RECIPES 194
CHAPTER 10: POULTRY RECIPE 208
CHAPTER 11: DESSERT RECIPES 222
CHAPTER 12: SIDE DISH 235
CHAPTER 13: SOUP AND SALAD 241
CHAPTER 14: MEAT DISH 247
CONCLUSION 258

STOPPING KIDNEY DISEASE (WITH 90+ RECIPES)

The power of renal diet to manage kidney disease, avoid dialysis with low sodium, low potassium, and low phosphorus recipes

Lewis W. Martin

THE STRUCTURE OF THE KIDNEY

The kidneys are two paired organs located on either side of the spine at about the level of the lower ribs.

Every healthy kidney is about 9 to 12 cm long, 4 to 6 cm wide and 3 to 5 cm thick, depending on the size of the human body. Together, the two kidneys weigh only about 300 g. The surface of healthy kidneys is usually smooth. Since they perform many tasks for the body, they are very well supplied with blood. About 1,800 liters of blood flow through the kidney daily.

In the renal cortex are many small blood vessel balls, the so-called glomeruli. In these glomeruli, the blood vessel wall is permeable to various components of the blood. While the blood cells, i.e. red and white blood cells, and plasma albumin (blood protein) cannot escape from the blood vessel, glucose (sugar), urea, electrolytes, and water pass through the vessel walls and are collected in the so-called tubules. The fluid collected in the tubules is called primary urine. Approx. 125 ml of primary urine are formed in this way every minute. This equates to almost 180 liters per day. The primary urine contains salts, nutrients, and slags, but no blood cells and no protein. Excretion via the kidneys is mainly ensured by two different mechanisms:

The tubules run meandering through the renal cortex and the medulla adjacent to the middle of the kidney. In this way, many components of the primary urine and almost all the fluid are reabsorbed and remain with the body. This leads to a concentration of the primary urine; the result is the actual urine (urine). This contains, in a healthy kidney daily, about 20 to 30 g of urea, 0.25 to 0.75 g of uric acid, 0.5 to 1.8 g of creatinine and 0.7 to 1.5 g of phosphate.

In the body, the kidneys are responsible for:

- fluid and electrolyte balance
- the regulation of blood pressure
- detoxification, as well as regulation of urea and creatinine

- the regulation of the acid-base household
- the regulation of red blood cell formation as well
- the production of hormones and enzymes

Chronic kidney disease usually progresses slowly. With the help of blood and urine examinations, it is possible to estimate whether the kidneys are still working adequately or, for example, dialysis should be started soon.

Blood and urine tests are not only necessary to detect chronic kidney disease. Also, in the further course, regular controls are very important: They show if and if so, how fast the illness progresses and help to estimate the risk of complications. Depending on the stage of the disease, the therapy can be adapted individually, and the next treatment steps can be discussed and planned in good time with the doctor. This is important, for example, when it is foreseeable that dialysis will be necessary.

CHRONIC KIDNEY FAILURE

Chronic renal failure (renal insufficiency) causes a deterioration of renal function. This increases the concentration of urinary substances in the blood (substances that have to be eliminated via the kidneys), e.g. creatinine and urea. The regulation of the water, electrolyte and acid-base balance is impaired. After the kidney forms hormones or activates vitamins, it can, among other things, lead to disorders of blood formation and changes in bone metabolism.

The kidneys can be damaged by inflammatory processes, vascular changes and various other diseases (high blood pressure, diabetes mellitus, and genetic factors). Chronic kidney disease develops over months or years; usually, both kidneys are affected.

Which stages can the disease go through?

Chronic kidney disease is divided into five stages:

Stage 1: Urinalysis shows signs of kidney damage. Healthy areas of the kidneys, however, ensure that they still function as normal.

Stage 2: In addition to kidney damage, kidney function is also slightly limited. Usually, however, no symptoms are noticeable.

Stage 3: Kidney function is moderately limited.

Stage 4: Kidney function is severely limited. There may already be episodes such as itching, anemia, hyperacidity or bone pain.

Stage 5: Terminal Renal Failure: The kidneys can no longer sufficiently cleanse the blood - there is often pronounced uremia. A dialysis or kidney transplant is needed to restore kidney function.

The health consequences of chronic kidney disease also depend on the state of health. Therefore, doctors are also investigating what could accelerate the progression of kidney failures - such as heart disease, a poorly adjusted high blood pressure or diabetes mellitus.

This is important to adapt the medication therapy individually - or to plan further steps with sufficient lead: For example, if you have a high risk that your kidneys will fail in the foreseeable future, you can discuss the treatment with the doctor as soon as possible. Perhaps more close follow-up examinations will be necessary.

WHAT ARE THE CAUSES OF CHRONIC KIDNEY FAILURE?

The triggers for chronic renal failure are mainly various diseases in question, for example:

Diabetes Mellitus: This is responsible for 40 per cent of all cases of chronic renal failure (diabetic nephropathy). High blood glucose levels in the long term damage the walls of the blood vessels and the other filter structures in the kidneys, making them more permeable to small protein particles, especially albumin. These are increasingly excreted in the urine. Also, a decline in filter particles (glomeruli) leads to a progressive reduction in detoxification performance.

Inflammation of the filter particles in the renal corpuscles (glomerulonephritis, but also systemic diseases such as lupus erythematosus): Approximately every fourth chronic renal insufficiency is caused among other things by immune and autoimmune reactions, infectious diseases or tumors.

Cystic kidney and other genetic disorders: This congenital malformation causes about eight percent of all cases of chronic renal failure. The kidney function is restricted, e.g. by fluid-filled cavities (cysts).

Hypertension: Increased blood pressure damages the glomeruli and blood vessels in the kidney over time. Paradoxically, in kidney disease increased blood pressure, more hormones are formed and less fluid is excreted. Impaired kidney function and hypertensive condition mutually reinforce each other.

Diseases of the blood vessels, e.g. atherosclerosis: may lead to reduced renal blood flow.

Medicines: The kidneys filter drugs and their breakdown products from the blood. Some substances can damage the kidney tissue, e.g. certain antibiotics, analgesics, and cytostatics.

WHAT SYMPTOMS CAN OCCUR?

Chronic kidney disease is often insidious and causes very different symptoms depending on the stage of the disease. In the beginning, there are usually no or only slight complaints. Only in case of a rapid deterioration of renal function can the first signs of illness already occur, e.g.:

- Increased excretion of light urine,
- High blood pressure,
- Edema in the legs, but also other parts of the body (e.g. eyelids),
- Red-colored urine (through the blood), foaming urine (through protein admixture).
- Greater renal impairment may, among other things, cause the following symptoms:
- Symptoms of anemia, such as skin blanching, feeling cold,

tiredness, weakness,
- Concentration and memory disorders,
- decreasing physical capacity,
- Nausea,
- Vomiting,
- Diarrhea,
- Itching and burning in the legs,
- Muscle and bone pain.

In the advanced stage, almost all organ systems are impaired by the lack of detoxification function of the kidneys. Typical end-stage symptoms (terminal kidney failure) include:

- Non-adjustable hypertension,
- The decrease in the amount of urine,
- Water retention
- Shortness of breath,
- Nausea,
- Vomiting,
- loss of appetite,
- irregular heartbeat,
- Drowsiness, drowsiness,
- Cramps,
- Coma.

MAIN CAUSES & RISK FACTORS

Common causes of chronic kidney failure are diabetes mellitus and high blood pressure, which account for about 35% of all cases. 15% of renal insufficiency patients suffer from inflammatory diseases of the renal corpuscles, the so-called glomerulonephritis. Hereditary diseases such as cystic kidney (8%) and kidney-damaging drugs or chronic renal pelvic inflammatory disease (5% each) are other causes. The various diseases lead to different rates of decline in kidney function.

Blood sugar and blood pressure significantly influence the

development and progression of chronic renal failure. Even a slight increase in blood pressure can speed kidney weakness along with diabetes. The systolic pressure in healthy people is in the range of 110-130 mmHg, the diastolic pressure is 70-80 mmHg. A pressure of 140/90 and above is considered elevated blood pressure.

However, the reasons for chronic kidney failure are not always known. There seems to be a genetic predisposition, as people with kidney-related relatives are also more likely to get kidney disease. In addition, we know today that obesity and smoking can increase the risk of chronic kidney failure.

Diabetes

The common cause of chronic kidney failure is diabetes. If the blood sugar level increases for a long time, there is a risk of chronic kidney disease. Increased blood sugar permanently damages the walls of the blood vessels. This hinders the blood flow and thus the nutrient transport to the organs. The late damage of diabetes in the kidneys is called diabetic nephropathy.

By damaging the small blood vessels in the kidneys, their wall becomes more permeable. Small protein particles, called albumins, slip through the vessel walls and are excreted in the urine. The detection of albumin in the urine is the first warning sign that diabetes causes damage to the kidneys. The narrowing of the small blood vessels in the kidneys also means that the kidney tissue is no longer sufficiently supplied with oxygen and nutrients, and the kidney cells die off.

Glomerulonephritis

The renal corpuscles are the "microfilters" of the kidneys and are also called glomeruli, which consist of tiny, coiled-up blood vessels that filter salts, metabolites, pollutants and, most importantly, fluid from the blood. Each kidney has about half to one million glomeruli contaminants in the blood that can cause the cells of the kidneys to become inflamed. Inflammations always affect both kidneys and, more or less, all kidney bodies.

Polycystic kidney disease

This congenital renal malformation usually leads to renal

insufficiency from the age of 40 years. Numerous fluid-filled cavities (cysts) restrict the function of kidney tissue. In childhood, these cysts are small, fill up more and more in the course of life with fluid and then displace the normal kidney tissue. This leads to renal insufficiency, which often leads to dialysis in the sixth decade of life.

High blood pressure
High blood pressure can both be the cause and consequence of chronic kidney weakness. On the one hand, high blood pressure damages the kidney bodies (glomeruli), so that they gradually fail. On the other hand, with decreasing renal function increased blood pressure, increasing hormones are formed. In addition, there is too much salt and water in the body, which also raises blood pressure.

Impaired kidney function and high blood pressure condition and reinforce each other. In many cases, hypertensive patients are, therefore, also kidney patients at the same time and vice versa.

Drugs
As an important excretory organ of the body, the kidneys also filter many drugs or their degradation products. However, some of these substances can damage kidney tissue. Medication-related kidney damage is generally rare and can occur only at very high doses (e.g. acetaminophen, see below) or in patients with certain risks. Medications that can occasionally cause such kidney damage include:

- Painkillers, such as paracetamol, ibuprofen, diclofenac
- Antibiotics, such as B. aminoglycosides (amikacin, gentamycin, neomycin or streptomycin)
- Anticancer drugs (chemotherapeutics)
- Iodinated contrast media.

Over-the-counter painkillers can cause kidney damage if taken for long periods. Thus, the active ingredient paracetamol from a total dose of 1,000 grams has a kidney-damaging effect - an amount that is achieved with the twice-daily intake of 500-milligram tablets after three years. Also, in the long-term use of pantoprazole and other blockers of gastric acid (so-called PPIs), kidney damage is increasingly being discussed recently.

Improper use or wrong dosage of even hypertension and diuretic drugs (diuretics) may trigger a more acute renal failure.

Diseases of the blood vessels

Chronic diseases of the blood vessels can impair kidney function. Vascular diseases can lead to reduced blood flow and thus trigger reduced blood flow to the kidneys. If there are deposits of lime and fats (so-called plaques) on the vessel wall, as is the case with arteriosclerosis, the vessels can gradually close completely, so that the underlying kidney tissue is no longer supplied with blood and dies. This can also affect blood vessels that are outside the kidneys. For example, if there is a constriction between the abdominal aorta and the kidney, this is called renal artery stenosis.

Blood vessels can also become inflamed; this is called vasculitis (from the Latin vas for blood vessel). Such vasculitis sometimes occurs only at the kidney, more often the kidney and other organs are affected. They often run very fast, i.e. kidney function can be completely lost within weeks. Fortunately, the doctors have very good medicines to cure vascular inflammation, at least in case of a timely diagnosis.

CHRONIC KIDNEY WEAKNESS: FIRST SIGNS & SYMPTOMS

First signs
The beginning of a chronic kidney weakness is often marked only by low signs of disease or even runs completely symptom-free. Often the kidney problems are superimposed by the symptoms of the underlying disease, such as the symptoms of diabetes or vasculitis.

Early symptoms of kidney disease can be:

- Increased excretion of less colored, light urine
- Increased blood pressure
- Water retention (edema) on the legs, around the eyes or all over the body
- Red urine.

Symptoms
A gradual course with little or no discomfort is characteristic of chronic renal insufficiency. An initially occurring high blood pressure of over 140/90 mmHg or an increasingly difficult to set high blood pressure can be an early sign of disease.

Many patients often produce bright, low-concentration urine and store water in the skin and subcutaneous tissue (edema). Foaming urine when urinating may be an indication of protein in the urine. A healthy kidney excretes at most 200 milligrams of protein per day, of which at most 30 milligrams of the blood protein albumin. At higher values, one speaks of microalbuminuria, starting from 300 milligrams albumin per day of proteinuria. Some patients also excrete blood with the urine. If this occurs in larger quantities, the urine is colored red (gross hematuria). Most of the time, however, there is only so little blood in the urine that it is invisible to the naked eye and can only be recognized by test strips (microhematuria).

With the progressive loss of function, the kidneys can no longer fulfill their tasks. It comes to disturbances of the water balance, the acid-base and the electrolyte balance and other organ systems. Also, the body is more susceptible to infections. Since the kidneys no longer produce sufficient amounts of the hematopoietic hormone erythropoietin (EPO), the number of red blood cells decreases. Such anemia leads to fatigue, weakness, difficulty concentrating and decreasing exercise capacity.

A noticeable paleness of the skin is another possible clinical indication. Besides, patients often experience nausea, vomiting, or diarrhea shortly before starting dialysis. Other symptoms may include memory impairment, itching and burning in the legs and muscle and bone pain.

In the advanced stage of chronic renal failure, almost all organ systems are damaged by the lack of detoxification function of the kidneys (uremic syndrome). There are abnormal changes in the cardiovascular system, the hematopoietic system, the gastrointestinal tract, the peripheral and central nervous system, the skin, the hormone system, and the bones.

Typical symptoms of end-stage renal failure (terminal kidney failure) are:

- Unacceptable high blood pressure
- Decrease in urine output
- Water retention (edema)
- shortness of breath
- Nausea, vomiting, loss of appetite
- Irregular heartbeat
- Drowsiness
- Convulsions, coma.

With the help of the so-called Glomerular Filtration Rate (GFR), chronic renal insufficiency is divided into five stages. The GFR is a laboratory value that is 90-130 milliliters per minute for normally functioning kidneys. This means that a healthy kidney purifies at least 90 milliliters of blood from freely filterable substances per minute and excretes them via the urine.

Stage I: GFR greater than 90 milliliters/ minute

Patients often have no symptoms at this stage. The blood levels for creatinine are still normal, only the protein excretion via the urine may be increased, or there are other indications, for example, as in the ultrasound, a kidney disease. If possible causes are already recognized, a worsening of the disease can very often still be prevented.

Stage II: GFR between 60-89 milliliters/ minute

Even at this stage, the kidney weakness is often not yet seen by blood tests. The kidneys still seem to function adequately, but more detailed studies show kidney disease, for example, with the measurement of urine protein or ultrasound. In addition, more accurate measurements, such as creatinine clearance, can detect a beginning of kidney failure.

Stage III: GFR between 30-59 milliliters/ minute

Renal damage has now progressed so fast that elevated creatinine and urea levels are also measured in the blood. Those affected suffer from high blood pressure, reduced performance, and faster fatigue. In stage III, the risk of cardiovascular disease increases significantly. The symptoms allow for different interpretations and do not necessarily indicate kidney weakness. Medicines that are normally excreted through the kidneys must now be reduced in their dose, so they do not cause any side effects.

Stage IV: GFR between 15-29 milliliters/ minute

At this stage, so many kidney cells are already defective that the deficient elimination of toxins affects the entire organism. The symptoms, therefore, increase the loss of appetite, tiredness, vomiting, nausea, nerve pain, itching, and bone pain. Because the body excretes fewer salts and water, it also leads to edema.

Stage V: GFR below 15 milliliters/ minute

If the kidney function is severely limited or the kidneys are eliminated, it is also called end-stage renal failure. The blood must be regularly cleaned at this stage by a blood wash (dialysis) of toxins. Otherwise, the body is poisoned. In spite of regular blood lavage, terminal renal insufficiency may still result in a yellowish discoloration of the skin and itching of the skin. Both are due to the deposition of substances in the skin, which would have to be excreted via the urine.

KIDNEY WEAKNESS (CHRONIC): EFFECTS & COMPLICATIONS

Disorders of blood purification, as well as the water and salt balance, affect many other organs of the body. Chronic renal insufficiency can, therefore, lead to various complications:

High blood pressure
An important consequence of a chronic renal failure is increased blood pressure: About 80% of the so-called kidney patients suffer from it. However, high blood pressure can also be the cause of kidney weakness. With decreasing urine output, the body cannot get rid of excess salt and water, which raises blood pressure. In addition, this leads to fluid retention, especially in the legs (edema). In extreme cases, fluid accumulates in the lungs, causing coughing with whitish to foamy secretions and severe shortness of breath (pulmonary edema).

Heart failure, cardiac arrhythmia, heart attack, stroke

In addition, there is further damage in the cardiovascular system, in particular to a pronounced calcification of arteries and also heart valves. Thus, valvular heart disease or heart failure occurs as a result of chronic kidney failure, and of course, heart attack and stroke through the calcified arteries. The kidneys increasingly lose the ability to regulate potassium in kidney failure, especially with a daily urine volume of less than one liter, the potassium levels in the blood can rise (hyperkalemia), which is characterized by a slowed heartbeat, dizziness and short loss of consciousness as well as muscle weakness and tingling sensations. Cardiac arrhythmias threaten cardiac arrest in greatly increased potassium levels. The excess water can also lead to a heart attack or stroke.

Disorders of the nervous system
Neurological disorders are also a common complication of advanced chronic renal failure. They can be measured as slowed nerve conduction velocity and altered brain waves in the electroencephalogram (EEG).

Possible symptoms are:

- Fatigue, memory and concentration disorders
- Optical hallucinations, disorientation, coma
- Itching, burning, muscle cramps or muscle weakness
- cognitive disorders
- sleep disorders
- anemia.

As kidney function weakens, lower levels of the hematopoietic hormone erythropoietin are also produced. This leads to anemia, the so-called renal anemia, which can manifest itself through increased fatigue, a striking pallor of the skin and declining physical resilience.

Disorders of bone metabolism
As renal function decreases, less active vitamin D is available to the body. Active vitamin D is a hormone that promotes the absorption of calcium via the intestine and the strength of the bones. If in the kidney, too little active vitamin D is formed, then the calcium content in the bone decreases, there are more fractures and more bone, muscle and joint pain. In addition, since the damaged kidneys excrete less phosphate, the phosphate level in the blood increases, which additionally promotes decalcification of the bones and the calcification of the arteries.

High phosphate levels in the blood cause itching, bone pain, and muscle aches. In addition, the increased accumulation in the body increases the risk of arteriosclerosis. This increases the risk of heart attack and stroke.

Malnutrition
Disturbances in protein and energy metabolism, hormonal imbalances, as well as nausea and loss of appetite are the reasons why many kidney disease patients are malnourished, especially when

protein metabolism is affected. Thus, the body absorbs fewer proteins with decreasing kidney function, and thus the calorie intake can go down.

PREGNANCY & KIDNEY WEAKNESS

Chronic kidney failure is more likely to result in premature birth, death of the unborn child, or birth defects. Complications of the mother may include bleeding, coagulation disorders, and hypertension. The risk, however, varies individually. Pregnant women with kidney disease must, therefore, be cared for by experienced doctors.

If the creatinine level in the blood is significantly increased, a viable child is rarely born. In normal creatinine, the higher the amount of protein in the urine, the more problematic the pregnancy. In about 5-10% of first-time mothers, urine protein is increased towards the end of pregnancy. A combination of increased urinary protein increases blood pressure and water retention in the tissue (edema), this is called gestosis.

Water retention can occur in any pregnancy. This explains a lot of the weight gain. After delivery, this fluid is excreted again, and the mother loses the extra body weight. Sometimes, however, stronger edema accumulates. These are disturbing but not dangerous, as long as there is no protein in the urine, and the blood pressure remains normal. In this case, the doctor can treat the water retention with leg elevation, less salt consumption, and support stockings. On the other hand, diuretics should not be given during pregnancy as they can slow down the flow of blood to the mother cake.

Kidney weakness (chronic): examinations & diagnosis
Many kidney diseases lead to long-lasting, irreversible kidney tissue damage. In contrast to acute renal failure, timely treatment can, in most cases, lead to stabilization or even recovery of renal function. The medical history of the patient and the physical examination play an important role.

For his diagnosis, the doctor must know about pre-existing kidney damage, chronic illnesses, and taking medications. Also, evidence of kidney disease in the family of the person affected is important.

The measurement of blood pressure and heart rate as well as the condition of the skin and the filling of the jugular veins allow conclusions on the fluid balance and thus on a possible water overload. With a 24-hour blood pressure measurement, the doctor can determine whether a patient has a normal blood pressure during the day, but suffers from unnoticed nocturnal hypertension. This is common in diabetics. Lack of nocturnal drop in blood pressure significantly increases the risk of organ damage.

By means of an ultrasound examination, the kidney size and the condition of the kidney tissue can be determined. If the kidneys are very small, this is an indication of long-standing kidney damage.

Blood test
When the kidneys are unable to filter the blood adequately, creatine and urea accumulate in the blood. The doctor can control this by analyzing blood levels. The more creatinine and urea in the blood, the weaker the kidney filter function. The creatinine normal is 8-12 milligrams per liter of blood, the normal urea concentration in the blood between 200 and 450 milligrams per liter. As an alternative to creatinine, cystatin C in the blood is measured as the control value, but so far, this is not yet a routine examination.

The concentration of creatinine in the blood is used in routine clinical practice for a preliminary assessment of renal function. However, this is not very accurate for all people, as the creatinine level often increases only when renal function has dropped by almost half. Thus, a slight restriction of kidney function can be overlooked.

More suitable for an early diagnosis is the so-called creatinine clearance, which indicates how quickly the kidneys can filter out creatinine from the blood. For this, urine must be collected for 24 hours and creatinine in the blood and urine is determined at the same time. Reduced creatinine clearance is found before the rise of creatinine in the blood and can, therefore, early indicate damage to the kidneys. In addition, the physician calculates the glomerular filtration rate from creatinine in blood serum or another small substance in the blood, cystatin C.

In addition, the doctor will determine the number of white blood cells and other blood levels, such as C-reactive protein, liver values, and fat levels. The C-reactive protein is increasingly produced during inflammatory processes in the liver and can indicate the course of renal insufficiency. Along with the blood picture, which has increased white blood cells in inflammatory processes, can be found next to the medical history, evidence of inflammation in the body.

The measurement of calcium, phosphate, vitamins and parathyroid hormone provides information about a disturbed electrolyte balance and possible damage to the bones.

Urinalysis
Since there is usually little or no protein in the urine, urinary excretion of protein is an important indicator of the presence of kidney disease. For this purpose, the urine is collected and analyzed for over 24 hours. Alternatively, the physician can determine the ratio of protein to creatinine in the urine. In a healthy kidney, the filter tissue is so dense that no more than 200 milligrams of protein per day is excreted in the urine. Regular measurements of protein excretion are also an important part of monitoring disease progression, as more and more protein is detected in the urine as the disease progresses.

A rapid urine test with a test strip allows the doctor to make an initial assessment of kidney disease. The test strips measure the protein content and the blood cells in the urine. If the test result is conspicuous, the urine must be further tested for the type and amount of these proteins and cells. The so-called glomerular filtration rate (GFR) is another laboratory value by which the doctor can detect chronic urinary weakness early in the urine. With their help, he can assess the severity of the disease. The normal value of the glomerular filtration rate for creatinine is 90-130 milliliters per minute. That is, a healthy kidney purifies at least 90 milliliters of blood per minute. In a microscopic examination of the urine, the so-called urine sediment, the doctor looks for red and white blood cells. If there is evidence of damage to the renal corpuscles, it may be necessary to perform a puncture of the kidney for tissue collection and examination.

CHRONIC RENAL INSUFFICIENCY: TREATMENT

Untreated chronic renal insufficiency often leads after years to a complete failure of the kidneys (terminal kidney insufficiency), in particular with hereditary diseases of the kidneys or if much protein is present in the urine. The more treatment can reduce protein levels in the blood, the sooner it can prevent complete kidney failure.

The goal of any treatment is to prevent or at least delay the progression of the disease. Complete healing is not possible in most cases, but the sooner kidney failure is treated, the better the chances of success. In some hereditary diseases such as the familial cystic kidney, however, there is still no therapy.

One differentiates between the treatment of the disease, which is based on kidney weakness, such as diabetes, hypertension or glomerulonephritis, as well as asymptomatic treatment, which should mitigate the effects of renal insufficiency, such as anemia, edema, potassium increase. The early treatment of the underlying disease is a prerequisite for the successful treatment of renal insufficiency.

If kidney failure is not yet very advanced, it can be treated with medication. Later, usually, an artificial blood purification (dialysis) or kidney transplantation is required.

Medication
- Diabetes medications

In diabetes mellitus, blood-sugar-lowering drugs, antihypertensive agents for high blood pressure and anti-inflammatory drugs are used for inflammation of the renal corpuscles. A good blood sugar and blood pressure control and permanent control of these two values can prevent kidney disease from occurring in the first place or slow down the progression of existing kidney failure.

- Blood pressure medications

In hypertensive patients, antihypertensive agents may slow the progression of diminishing renal function. In this case, so-called ACE inhibitors and angiotensin II receptor antagonists are preferably used, which in addition to the blood pressure-lowering effect also hardly burden the kidneys. Significantly, the kidney-protective effect of ACE inhibitors is independent of blood pressure. Thus, the ACE inhibitors are also prescribed at normal blood pressure levels. The target value is a blood pressure of 130/80. To achieve this, in many cases, several drugs with different mechanisms of action must be used. Patients can support drug therapy through physical activity, not nicotine and low salt diet.

- Inflammation

Inflammation of the renal corpuscles (glomerulonephritis) can be treated with drugs that reduce the activity of the immune system. These so-called immunosuppressants include drugs, such as cortisone, cyclosporin or cyclophosphamide.

- Hormones

As renal insufficiency also reduces the formation of new red blood cells, in the case of anemia (renal anemia), the kidney hormone erythropoietin (Epo) is administered, which promotes blood formation and thus increases the number of red blood cells. Before using Epo, the doctor will measure the amount of iron in the body, as chronic kidney weakness and anemia often lack iron.

- Fat reducers

Blood lipid-lowering drugs, such as statins are used for the treatment of elevated cholesterol levels and the treatment of cardiovascular diseases such as arteriosclerosis.

- Diuretics and phosphate binders

Diuretic drugs, also known as diuretics, increase salt and water excretion. Although the drugs can increase the amount of urine, they do not improve the detoxification function of the kidneys. If a low-phosphate diet can no longer keep phosphate levels stable as the renal function progresses, so-called phosphate binders (calcium carbonate, potassium acetate, calcium citrate) are used. These bind some of the phosphates in the food already in the gastrointestinal tract. They should be taken in the correct dosage immediately before or at the beginning of the meal.

Treatment with vitamin D and/or vitamin D analogs also serves to normalize calcium and phosphate metabolism.

- Dialysis

According to current guidelines, the initiation of renal replacement therapy (dialysis) is recommended at the latest with a creatinine clearance of fewer than 5-10 milliliters/minute, in diabetes patients also earlier. If a patient is already suffering from damage to many organs (uremic syndrome), or if edema or high blood pressure can no longer be brought under control, kidney replacement therapy should also be started earlier.

The preparation and initiation of renal replacement therapy must be timely. An adequate nutritional status, a well-adjusted blood pressure, and a balanced blood count are important prerequisites.

If there is a terminal renal insufficiency despite all therapeutic measures, only dialysis or kidney transplant can help. This is the case when the consequences of impaired kidney function through an adapted diet and medication are no longer manageable. Since early-onset improves treatment prospects, preparations should begin in a good time. Today, there are two different blood purification methods: on the one hand hemodialysis as the most commonly used procedure and the other hand, peritoneal dialysis.

- Kidney transplant

In a kidney transplant, a kidney patient receives a healthy kidney from a living or deceased donor. The surgeon transplants the patient either a kidney from a dead or a living relative or close people. This is possible without health restrictions for the donor, because of the two kidneys, which each person usually owns. A single kidney is sufficient for blood purification and urine production.

The prerequisite for organ removal for a donation from a deceased person is the determination of brain death according to the German Transplantation Act, which came into force in 1997. In the case of a living donation, no economic motives or emotional constraints may influence the decision for the donation. The prerequisite is that the blood type and other specific genetic characteristics of donor and recipient match so that the recipient's immune system does not repel the new kidney.

DIET IN RENAL INSUFFICIENCY

Nutrition has a major impact on the treatment and disease course of kidney failure. Anyone who adheres to the recommendations of the doctors or dieticians, therefore, can significantly support the treatment of chronic renal insufficiency.

Acute renal insufficiency
Acute renal failure may lead to increased protein degradation and lipid metabolism disorders. Pay attention to your calorie intake. Recommended are 35 to 40 kilocalories per kilogram of body weight and day. Drink about as much as you left the day before. If the urine excretion is too low, patients should eat potassium, sodium and low protein. If the urine excretion is too high, a potassium and sodium-rich diet are recommended. This compensates for the loss of mineral salts. You can eliminate fluid loss by drinking enough.

CHRONIC RENAL INSUFFICIENCY

Chronic renal insufficiency: low protein diet
Reduced protein intake may appear to slow the progression of renal insufficiency. Therefore, you should not consume more than 0.6 to 0.8 grams of protein per kilogram of body weight per day.

The consumed protein should have a high biological value, i.e. consist of many protein building blocks, which the body cannot form itself (essential amino acids). The combination of different protein sources ensures the supply of all important compounds. Ideal protein mixtures include, for example, potato and egg, beans and egg, milk and wheat, egg and wheat, as well as legumes and wheat.

Also recommended is the use of low-protein specialty products such as low-protein flour and products made from it (bread, pastries).

Chronic renal insufficiency: a diet low in phosphate
Chronic renal insufficiency has negative effects on bone metabolism,

among other factors - bone stability decreases. In order not to increase this effect even further, a low-phosphate kidney diet is recommended, because too much phosphate makes the bones more brittle.

The recommended amount of phosphate is 0.8 to 1 gram per day. Restrict the consumption of high-phosphate foods. These include, for example, nuts, cereals, offal, and wholemeal bread. Many dairy products such as milk, yoghurt, and buttermilk also supply a lot of phosphates. Cheaper cheeses such as cottage cheese, cream cheese, Camembert, Brie, Mozzarella, Harzer Roller and Limburger are cheaper.

If possible, avoid foods with production-related phosphate additives such as processed cheese, cooked cheese, canned milk, and some sausages. You may want to ask about the phosphate content when buying sausages in the butchery. On the ingredient list of foods, you can see phosphate additives on the E numbers E 338 to E 341, E 450 a to c, E 540, E 543 and E 544. Incidentally, there is a close link between the phosphate and protein content - protein-rich foods usually also contain a lot of phosphates.

Chronic renal insufficiency: low potassium diet
Especially in the advanced stage of renal insufficiency, patients should eat low-potassium, so as not to increase the increased potassium due to renal insufficiency in the blood. Too much potassium can cause cardiac arrhythmias.

Depending on the severity of the kidney weakness, a potassium intake of 1.5 to 2 grams per day is recommended. The best way is to avoid potassium-rich foods and drinks. These include:

- Fruit and vegetable juices
- Dried fruit (raisins, dates, figs)
- nuts
- Bananas, apricots, avocado
- Pulses (peas, beans, lentils, etc.)
- Tomatoes, spinach, Swiss chard, broccoli, kale, Brussels sprouts, fennel, olives
- Sprouts and germs

- Mushrooms (fresh and dried)
- Potato dry products (potato chips, potato dumplings, and mashed potatoes)

Chronic renal insufficiency: the amount of drinking
Although many patients suspect the opposite: drinking a lot cannot improve kidney function. Rather, over-hydration can even accelerate the progression of chronic renal insufficiency. Talk to your doctor or dietician about how much fluids you should take daily.

Chronic renal insufficiency: diet on dialysis
Limited fluid intake is particularly important in patients whose chronic renal insufficiency necessitates dialysis treatment. Keeping a limited amount of fluid requires a lot of discipline. The daily amount of drinking depends on the urine excretion within 24 hours. As much fluid as you excrete, you should also reintroduce the body - plus about half a liter extra per day. Keep in mind, however, that you can cover some of your fluid requirements through your diet. Not only soups, but almost all foods contain water (for example, fruits, vegetables, yogurt, pudding, fish, and meat).

Tips for thirst-quenching:

- Chewing gum without sugar
- Suck ice cubes
- Lemon pieces suck
- Avoid salty and very sweet foods
- Rinse mouth

People with renal insufficiency who are on dialysis should control their weight daily. If the weight gain exceeds the level recommended by the physician, you should consult your doctor immediately.

NON-ALLOWED FOODS

To reduce sodium
- Broth nuts, meat extracts
- Foods in brine, in salt, in oil (capers, olives, meats or canned fish)

- Margarine, mayonnaise, mustard, other sauces
- Milk powder
- Savory snacks, peanuts, popcorn
- To reduce phosphorus
- Sausages in general and sliced meats
- Cheeses with the exception of ricotta and mozzarella
- Chocolate
- Brewer's yeast
- Offal (liver, kidney, heart, brain, etc.) and fatty meats: lamb, goose, duck, chicken, game.
- Egg yolk
- Dried vegetables
- Dried fruit
- Crayfish
- Flour
- Bran

To reduce potassium
The limitation of foods rich in potassium should be carried out only on the precise indication of the treating nephrologist, as many foods rich in potassium have important health values and can help prevent the onset of cardiovascular diseases so frequently associated with this disease.

- Grapefruit, bananas, chestnuts, coconuts, kiwi, dried fruit
- Fruit juices
- Artichokes and spinach
- Potatoes
- Bran
- Integral products
- Dietary salts
- legumes
- mushrooms
- Sausages
- Ham
- Soy
- Bitter cocoa and chocolate

- Milk powder
- Parsley
- Sardines, sardines, stockfish
- Brewer's yeast

FOODS ALLOWED WITH MODERATION

Salt: It is a good rule to reduce the amount added to the dishes during and after cooking and limit the consumption of foods that naturally contain high quantities (canned or brine foods, nuts, and meat extracts, soy-type sauces). Common salt should not be replaced with "dietary salts" because they are rich in potassium.

100 cc wine for lunch and 100 cc for dinner or 150 cc of beer for lunch and 150 cc for dinner, with the doctor's permission.

Coffee: Limit consumption, if the doctor does not completely forbid it, to two cups a day.

Honey, jam, and sugar: Although free of phosphorus, they must be consumed in moderation due to their simple sugar content.

To reduce sodium
- Pizza, bread, crackers, and breadsticks.
- To reduce phosphorus
- Milk, yogurt, cream
- Pasta, rice, barley
- Fresh legumes
- Chocolate
- Fish
- Fresh cheeses such as ricotta and mozzarella

ALLOWED AND RECOMMENDED FOODS

- Pasta, pana, rice.
- Tuscan bread. Tuscan bread can be replaced with breadsticks without salt or rusks without salt.

- Aproteic foods specially produced without proteins, which can improve the palatability of the diet such as bread, pasta, rice, flour, crackers, rusks, biscuits, and allow more acceptable portions of dishes that contain animal proteins. These foods are also available in supermarkets.
- Meat, all types except very fat ones. Choose the leanest and least veined parts. Poultry skin must be discarded.
- Fish, fresh or frozen except for fat varieties. Fresh fish must be washed in plenty of running water because sometimes it is stored in water and salt or under ice and salt before selling.
- Vegetables, both fresh and frozen, excluding legumes (beans, chickpeas, lentils, broad beans, peas). Mushrooms and artichokes can be eaten only occasionally.
- Fruit, with the exception of the aforementioned one, can be consumed either fresh or cooked, in a fruit salad or pureed without the addition of milk.
- Seasonings prefer the use of extra virgin olive oil or choose seed oil (not of various seeds but of a single seed, for example, corn oil, peanut oil, sunflower oil).
- Natural or mineral water.
- Spices and aromatic herbs.

BEHAVIORAL ADVICE

In the case of overweight or obesity, it is recommended to reduce the weight and the "waistline," which is the abdominal circumference, an indicator of the quantity of fat deposited on a visceral level. Waist circumference values greater than 94 cm in men and 80 cm in women are associated with a "moderate" cardiovascular risk, values greater than 102 cm in men and 88 cm in women are associated with a "high risk." Obesity is a cause of kidney failure.

Maintain an active lifestyle compatible with the degree of the illness (abandon sedentariness! Go to work on foot, by bicycle or park far away, if you can avoid the use of the elevator and take the stairs on foot).

Read the product labels, especially to ascertain their micronutrient content.

Adequate control of blood pressure. Maintain optimal blood pressure values by reducing the intake of salt and alcohol and/or using antihypertensive drugs.

Check body weight in the morning before breakfast. The increase of 1 kg of body weight or more in a short time (a few days), the appearance of swelling, or the reduction of diuresis, should not be underestimated, it should be referred to a specialist doctor.

If you are diabetic, check your blood sugar carefully.

Beware of drugs. Do not take anti-inflammatories without the advice of the nephrologist.

Not smoking. Smoking damages the kidneys.

PRACTICAL TIPS

To further reduce the amount of potassium in food, it is advisable to soak the vegetables and fruit in cold water 8-9 hours before consumption and boil them in abundant water.

To further reduce the amount of phosphorus in food, it is recommended to soak them in a container and keep them in the fridge 8-9 hours before cooking. Prefer cooking like boiling in plenty of water; it is also recommended to change it halfway through cooking.

SIMPLE NUTRITION TIPS

Less phosphorus
Phosphorus from food is absorbed in the intestine and excreted through the kidneys. If there is limited kidney function, this can lead to phosphate overload in the body. As a possible long-term consequence, particularly vascular calcifications, they must be feared. A low intake of phosphorus is hardly conceivable with a central European diet, as it is contained in many foods.

Particularly rich in phosphorus, for example, finished products, since the mineral is often part of a variety of additives. Melted cheese, for example, is one of the foods with extremely high phosphorus content due to its melting salts. One slice already covers a quarter of the maximum recommended amount in kidney failure. Meat, fish, eggs and dairy products should not be consumed in excessive quantities because of their content.

Phosphorus from plant sources such as whole-grain cereals, nuts or legumes is absorbed by the intestine to a much lesser extent and is, therefore, less of a problem.

Less sodium
Saline is the largest source of sodium in the western diet. The average Austrian usually eats about one third more saline than recommended. Ingesting too much salt through food may cause high blood pressure, over-hydration and, subsequently, left heart hypertrophy in patients with renal insufficiency. Like phosphorus, salt hides in considerable quantities in finished products, munchies, processed meat products, and cheese. A frozen pizza, for example, covers on average, three-quarters of the daily recommended maximum amount of table salt. Therefore, as far as possible, do not use finished products and do not salt them at the table.

Balanced ratio
To optimally support the metabolism with reduced kidney function, it can help to select the main nutrients protein, fat, and carbohydrates. Although protein is an important component of the body cell, however, too much animal protein - as is common in the general Austrian diet - can lead to increased acidity in the body. Especially the high consumption of meat and sausage ensures that the average Austrian absorbs about one third more protein than recommended. On the one hand, the most important measure should be to pay attention to small portion sizes and, on the other hand, to limit the frequency of consumption of animal protein carriers such as meat, poultry, eggs, sausages, and dairy products.

Particularly favorable is the combination of increased vegetables and fewer animal proteins. From the age of 65, the protein intake can be slightly increased again, as protein synthesis decreases with increasing age. The amount of ingested fat can basically be based on the situation of the person concerned. Due to the high energy value, it should be used sparingly in case of overweight. On the other hand, with the risk of malnutrition, increased fat intake can contribute to a good nutritional status.

Still fed up
To compensate for the smaller portion of meat, sufferers can eat plenty of complex carbohydrates and fiber. Vegetables, lettuce and carbohydrate-rich side dishes such as potatoes, rice, and noodles cause good satiety and have no negative impact on kidney function. This also applies to diabetics, if it is paid attention to, it is good for controlling blood sugar.

The currently very popular carbohydrate-reduced diets, in which precisely those supplements for weight loss are avoided, usually provide automatically for increased protein intake. Therefore, they are not suitable for people with chronic renal failure. Every day two hands full of fruit and plenty of vegetables - no matter in which form - supplement the diet with filling and digestive fiber as well as vitamins and minerals.

Rethinking dialysis
Once chronic kidney disease has become so advanced that renal replacement therapy in the form of hemodialysis or peritoneal dialysis becomes necessary, some of the nutritional needs of patients change. For example, a higher protein intake benefits the patients, but often the consumption of fruits and vegetables has to be limited. By that time at the latest, a detailed nutritional consultation by a doctor or dietician should take place.

DIETARY GUIDELINES

The following are some essential dietary guidelines concerning proteins, potassium restriction, phosphorus restriction, sodium restriction, and moisture restriction.

Protein
Proteins (= proteins) are the building blocks of the body and have different functions. They are essential for building muscle, providing protection against infections, ensuring the repair and renewal of cells in our body. A balanced intake of proteins through the diet must be sought. How many proteins are allowed daily depends on the remaining kidney function (no kidney replacement therapy) or the type of kidney replacement therapy (hemodialysis or peritoneal dialysis).

Proteins are broken down to urea, are then released into the blood as waste and are usually excreted by the kidneys. Proteins are found in many foods, but not always in the same amount. Meat, fish, cheese, eggs, dairy products, and soy contain high-quality proteins.

Bread, potatoes and grain products (rice, pasta, etc.) also contain proteins but to a lesser extent and of lesser quality, but these foods are indispensable as an energy source.

· If the kidneys function less well (= renal failure), but kidney replacement therapy is not yet required, it is essential that the protein intake through the diet does not rise too high.

The less well-functioning kidneys excrete fewer waste materials (including proteins). The proteins absorbed through the diet must be of good quality.

If kidney replacement therapy is already required, the daily protein intake through the diet is higher since dialysis causes an additional loss of protein. A protein deficiency would lead to muscle weakness, reduced resistance, malnutrition, etc. what should be prevented.

Phosphorus restriction
The terms phosphate and phosphorus are often used interchangeably.

Phosphorus accumulates in the blood if the kidneys not or insufficiently excrete it. Too much phosphorus in the blood can lead to bone loss, joint pains and itching. During dialysis, part of the phosphorus is removed from the blood. Part of this will also be removed via phosphate-binding medication prescribed by the doctor. However, these measures are often not sufficient, so that the intake of phosphorus via the diet must also be limited. Phosphorus is mainly found in foods that contain proteins. Protein-rich foods are, therefore, even phosphorus-rich foods. In addition to a lot of salt, most types of cheese also include a lot of phosphorus and are not recommended for people with kidney disease. Phosphorus is also used as an additive to soft drinks, which also have no nutritional value so that they are avoidable. A good knowledge of which foods contain phosphorus and the correct use of phosphate binders is essential here. Some tips regarding the use of phosphate binders:

- Take the phosphate binders during meals. The phosphate binders then come together with the food in the intestines. In this way, most of the phosphorus from the protein-rich meals can be bound.
- Also consider the protein-rich snacks such as yogurt, pudding, and cheese that are phosphor-rich because phosphate binders may then also be required.
- If you do not eat, for example, during illness, then naturally phosphate binders should not be taken.
- Phosphorus is mainly in the following foods:
- Whole grain products (wholemeal and brown bread, brown rice and pasta, muesli, whole grain breakfast cereals, dried fruit cereals)
- Meat, meat products, fish, meat substitutes, egg yolk
- Milk and milk products, cheese, cheese spread
- Certain types of vegetables: mainly artichoke, corn, mushrooms, and sprouts
- Certain types of fruit: dried fruit and passion fruit
- Products based on cocoa (chocolate, chocolate spread, cookies with chocolate, pralines, etc.)
- Nuts, seeds, seeds, legumes
- Cola, beer and lawyer.

Potassium restriction

Potassium is an essential mineral and helps the heart to function properly. Usually, the kidneys regulate the amount of potassium in the body. With reduced kidney function, the excess potassium is not removed and accumulates. Too high a potassium level in the blood can cause serious cardiac arrhythmias. The level of potassium in your blood can be reduced by restricting the use of potassium-rich foods. Potassium is mainly found in the following foods:

- Potatoes
- Whole-grain cereals (whole-grain and brown bread, brown rice and pasta, muesli, whole-grain breakfast cereals, dried cereal breakfast cereals)
- Vegetables, fruit and dried fruit
- Milk and milk products
- Certain drinks (strong coffee, fresh or ready-to-buy fruit, and vegetable juices
- Cocoa-based products (chocolate, chocolate spread, chocolate cookies, pralines, etc.)
- Nuts, seeds, seeds, and legumes
- Dietary products without salt and substitute salt.

Some facts and tips about potassium:

Potassium is soluble in water. When boiling vegetables and potatoes in plenty of water, about 1/3 of the potassium is lost if you discard the boiling water at the end of the boiling process and replace it with fresh boiling water (so-called "boiling in two times").

* Potatoes are particularly potassium-rich. Replacing the potatoes with white rice or white pasta a few times a week is a good habit. White rice and white pasta (spaghetti, spirelli, macaroni, tagliatelle, noodles, etc.) contain much less potassium compared to potatoes and are therefore good alternatives.

* When using vegetables rich in potassium, replace the portion of potatoes with a piece of white rice or white pasta.

* Coffee can be replaced by tea or soft drinks. These drinks hardly contain any potassium.

* Preparation method of potatoes and vegetables:

- Potatoes:

Always peel the potatoes, cut them into small pieces and boil them twice in water, throwing out the first boiling water. Finish with mash, baked potatoes, croquettes, etc. if necessary. Potatoes cooked in the peel lose practically no potassium and are therefore best avoided.

- Vegetables:

Clean the vegetables and cut them into small pieces. Boil the plants once in a generous amount of water. Then drain the cooking liquid. After all, there is a lot of potassium in this boiling fluid, and it should therefore not be used to prepare a sauce. Finish the greetings with a little fat if necessary.

* Avoid cooking in the microwave, in a steam device, in a pressure cooker or baking in the oven, wok. These cooking techniques can only be used to heat already cooked potatoes and vegetables.

Sodium restriction
Sodium is a mineral that occurs in the body and is indispensable for certain functions of the body, such as water management.

If the kidneys are still functioning normally, the excess of sodium will be discharged. If the kidneys no longer work optimally, too much sodium remains in the blood. Too much sodium in the blood and salt (= NaCl) in the diet leads to thirst, fluid retention and an increase in blood pressure.

Sodium is a natural component of salt (= NaCl). By salt, we mean table salt, sea salt, salt enriched with iodine,

If one is advised to use less salt (NaCl), then it is actually meant that one must limit the sodium through the diet. Sodium is naturally present in almost all foods. For example, potatoes and vegetables do not contain a small amount of sodium during the preparation without adding salt. For many foods, sodium is added extra during the production process in the factory.

Some tips on how to reduce salt intake:

- do not add extra salt when preparing the meal or at the table;
- limit the use of foods that are high in salt, such as:
    - Smoked fish and meat and imposed products;
    - Cheese, processed cheese, melted cheese;
    - Ready-made spice mixtures (e.g. for spaghetti, barbecue, salads), sauces, canned soups, instant soup;
    - Ready-made (frozen and fresh) meals, breaded meals (fish steaks, schnitzel), prepared frozen vegetables (e.g. leeks in cream sauce);
    - Seasonings, such as stock cubes, mustard, ketchup, soy sauce.
    - Salty snacks such as salty peanuts, crisps, aperitif cookies, cheese.
    - Solid cheeses and French cheeses contain more salt compared to cheeses such as flat cheeses, cottage cheese, mozzarella, ricotta, ...;
- Use other flavorings instead of salt, such as fresh herbs, spices, onion, garlic, lemon, etc. An herbal guide can help with this.
- Finish a dish with a twist of the pepper mill;
- Meat and fish can be seasoned well in a marinade (without salt);
- Unprepared frozen foods (vegetables, meat, fish, etc.) do not contain any added salt;
- Always give preference to fresh products (vegetables, meat, fish, etc.);
- Sea salt and iodine-enriched salt contain as much sodium as common kitchen salt;
- Preferably use low-salt bread or unsalted rusks;
- If the bread itself is baked, add less salt;
- Prefer fish and meat preparations in papillote and roasting. The taste is better preserved.
- DO NOT use substitute salt or diet products with less salt (low-salt cheeses, low-salt meats).

CAUTION FOR "DIET SALT" or

"REPLACEMENT SALT"

These products often contain less or no sea salt, but sodium is often replaced by potassium which is not suitable for a potassium restriction! Moreover, this way, you maintain poor habituation to the salty taste.

Humidity limitation

A certain amount of fluid is necessary for everyone since our body consists of approximately 2/3 of water. Normally, an excess of ingested fluid is removed by the kidneys. With impaired renal function, fluid accumulates in the body, resulting in fluid retention (edema), feeling tight and increased blood pressure. All these can be prevented provided that there is an adjusted (limited) fluid intake (individually). The amount of fluid that can still be used daily depends, among other things, on the remaining urine production and is calculated according to the amount of urine that is still formed in 24 hours.

The permitted drink per day = 500 ml to 750 ml PLUS the number of ml urine output in 24 hours. The drink includes not only water, but also coffee, tea, soft drinks, soup, milk, custard, sauce, fruit juice or vegetable juice, etc. In addition, solid foods naturally also bring in a certain amount of moisture. For example, vegetables, fruit, and potatoes consist of 90% water.

The total amount of moisture that is added daily by the solid foods is approximately 500 ml. These are not included in the permitted amount of drink per day (500 ml to 750 ml). A few tips to better maintain

Your fluid restriction:

- spread your fluid intake throughout the day;
- Use small cups, small glasses, etc. to distribute the amount of moisture better;
- Drink with small nibs and prefer fresh, not too sweet drinks;
- At parties, it is best to choose drinks that are served in small quantities (sherry, (foam) wine, champagne, spirits such as whiskey, cognac, etc. but in moderation) instead of soft drinks,

beers, cocktails, ...;
- To avoid feeling thirsty, it is best to avoid as many salt-rich, sugar-rich and highly spiced (spicy) foods as possible;
- Take your medication with the meal or dessert (e.g. pudding, yogurt, etc.) or with the drink with the meal;
- If you still feel thirsty, use a slice of lemon to moisten your lips, add an ice cube with possibly some lemon juice for an even fresher taste and increase saliva production (corresponds to 15 ml of water). You can also use a small portion of the fruit that you could freeze for this. You can also rinse the mouth with water.
- The use of humidifiers can also be a tool to prevent dry mouth and provide the necessary refreshment in hot weather.

TOP 15 KIDNEY-FRIENDLY NUTRITION FOR PEOPLE WITH KIDNEY PROBLEMS

1. Red pepper
- 75 grams of red pepper = 1 mg of sodium, 88 mg of potassium, 10 mg of phosphorus

Red peppers have a low potassium value and have a lot of taste, but that is not the only reason why they fit well in a kidney-friendly diet. These tasty vegetables are an excellent source for vitamin C, vitamin A. Vitamin B6, folic acid and fiber. Red peppers are good for you because they contain lycopene, an antioxidant that protects you against cancer.

2. Cabbage
- 75 grams of green cabbage = 6 mg of sodium, 60 mg of potassium and 9 mg of phosphorus

Cabbage is a cruciferous vegetable and is packed with phytochemicals, chemical components in fruit or vegetables that neutralize free radicals before they can cause damage. Many phytochemicals are known to fight cancer and to support cardiovascular health.

Cabbage contains a lot of vitamin K, vitamin C, and fiber. It is also a good source of vitamin B6 and folic acid. It is low in potassium and inexpensive and is, therefore, an affordable addition to a kidney-friendly diet.

3. Cauliflower
- 75 grams of cooked cauliflower = 9 mg of sodium, 88 mg of potassium and 20 mg of phosphorus

Cauliflower, another cruciferous vegetable, is a good source of vitamin C, fiber and folate (one of the B vitamins, and in large quantities also called folic acid and vitamin B9). It is also full of indoles, glucosinolates, and thiocyanates - constituents that help the liver neutralize toxins that damage cell membranes and DNA.

4. Garlic
- 1 clove of garlic = 1 mg of sodium, 12 mg of potassium and 4 mg of phosphorus

Garlic helps to prevent plaque, lowers your cholesterol and reduces inflammation.

5. Onions
- 75 grams of onions = 3 mg of sodium, 116 mg of potassium and 3 mg of phosphorus

Onions are part of the basic flavorings in every kitchen, contain sulfur, and therefore give it its sharp odor. Although onions make some people shed tears, they are also rich in flavonoids, and in particular quercetin, a powerful antioxidant that helps fight heart disease and protects against various cancers. Onions are low in potassium and are a good source for chromium, a mineral that helps in carbohydrate, protein and fat metabolism.

6. Apples
- 1 medium apple with zest = 0 sodium, 158 mg of potassium and 10 mg

Apples are known to lower cholesterol, prevent constipation, protect against heart disease and reduce the risk of cancer. Apples are high in fiber and have many anti-inflammatory components. The slogan "Sweets healthy, eat an apple" seems to have a solid foundation.

7. Cranberries
- 75 grams of cranberry juice cocktail = 3 mg of sodium, 22 mg of potassium and 3 mg of phosphorus

- 40 grams of cranberry sauce = 35 mg of sodium, 17 mg of potassium and 6 mg of phosphorus

- 75 grams of dried cranberries = 2 mg of sodium, 24 mg potassium, and 5 mg phosphorus

These tasty berries are known to offer protection against bladder infection by preventing bacteria from sticking to the bladder wall. Similarly, cranberries protect the stomach from ulcer-causing bacteria, and protect your gastrointestinal tract and even help improve its health. It has also been found that cranberries help against cancer and heart disease.

8. Blueberries
- 75 grams of fresh blueberries = 4 mg of sodium, 75 mg of potassium and 7 mg of phosphorus

Blueberries contain many antioxidant phytonutrients called anthocyanidins, which give them their blue color. They are full of natural compounds that reduce inflammation. Blueberries are a good source of vitamin C, manganese (that keeps your bones healthy), and fiber. They can also help protect your brain against some of the effects of aging.

9. Raspberries
- 75 grams of raspberries = 0 mg of sodium, 93 mg of potassium and 7 mg of phosphorus

Raspberries contain a phytonutrient called ellagic acid that helps neutralize free radicals in the body and thus prevent cell damage. They also contain the flavonoids anthocyanins - antioxidants that give raspberries their red color. Raspberries are an excellent source for manganese, vitamin C, fiber and folate, a vitamin B. Raspberries can have properties that can prevent cancer cell growth and tumor formation.

10. Strawberries
- 75 grams (5 medium) fresh strawberries = 1 mg of sodium, 120 mg of potassium and 13 mg of phosphorus

Strawberries are full of two types of phenols: anthocyanins and ellagitannins. Anthocyanins give strawberries their red color and are powerful antioxidants that help protect the structure of body cells and prevent damage due to oxidation. Strawberries are full of vitamin C and manganese and are an excellent source of fiber. They are known to protect the heart and contain anti-cancer and anti-inflammatory properties.

11. Cherries
75 grams of fresh (sweet) cherries = 0 mg of sodium, 160 mg of sodium and 15 mg of phosphorus

Eating cherry daily helps prevent inflammation. They are also full of antioxidants and phytochemicals that protect the heart.

12. Red Grapes
- 75 grams of red grapes = 1 mg of sodium, 88 mg of potassium and 4 mg of phosphorus

Red grapes contain different flavonoids that give them their reddish color. Flavonoids prevent oxidation and reduce blood clots and thereby help protect against heart disease. Resveratol, a flavonoid contained in grapes, can also stimulate the production of nitrogen oxides; this helps relax the muscle cells in blood vessels and promote blood flow. These flavonoids also protect against cancer and prevent inflammation.

13. Protein
- 2 proteins = 7 grams of protein, 110 mg of sodium, 108 mg of potassium and 10 mg of phosphorus

Protein is pure protein and provides the highest amount of protein with all essential amino acids. Proteins fit well in a kidney-friendly diet because they contain less phosphorus than other proteins such as egg yolk or meat.

14. Fish
- 85 grams of wild salmon = 50 mg of sodium, 368 mg of potassium and 274 mg of phosphorus

Fish supplies high-quality protein and contains omega 3, an anti-inflammatory fat. These healthy fats in fish help to combat diseases such as heart disease and cancer. Omega 3 also helps in lowering LDL cholesterol (the bad cholesterol) and in raising HDL, the good variant of cholesterol. Fish species high in omega 3 include Albine tuna, herring, mackerel, rainbow trout, and salmon.

15. Olive oil
- 1 tablespoon of olive oil = less than 1 mg of sodium, less than 1 mg

of potassium and 0 mg of phosphorus

Olive oil is a great source of oleic acid, a fatty acid with an anti-inflammatory effect. The unsaturated acid in olive oil protects against oxidation. Olive oil is rich in polyphenols and antioxidants that prevent inflammation and oxidation.

Research shows that populations that use large amounts of olive oil instead of other oils are less likely to suffer from heart disease and cancer.

Virgin or extra virgin olive oil contains more antioxidants.

TIPS TO PREVENT KIDNEY DAMAGE

Tips for a healthy lifestyle
Maintaining a healthy lifestyle sounds so simple, but it is sometimes so difficult. Below you can read what a healthy lifestyle is and how you can reduce the risk of kidney damage. Many of these recommendations will correspond to the lifestyle recommendations that are given for high blood pressure and diabetes, diseases that in themselves can lead to kidney damage.

Healthy food
Whoever eats according to the guidelines of the Voedingscentrum and also has a regular eating pattern, will feel nice and fit and also reduce the risk of kidney damage. Eat varied, not too much, less saturated fat, less salt, lots of vegetables, lots of fruit and enough bread.

Healthy weight
People who are overweight have an increased risk of kidney damage (and of other diseases such as diabetes and cardiovascular disease). It is, therefore, important to strive for a healthy weight. The Body Mass Index (BMI) is used worldwide to determine whether someone has a healthy weight. So check regularly how your BMI is doing.

Enough exercise
For your health, it is useful to moderate intensity for one hour daily exercise. That means that you have to breathe correctly, and your heart beats faster. Moving for half an hour does not have to be consecutive.

Cycling twice for 15 minutes or walking ten times for 10 minutes is also possible.

Do not smoke
Smoking can damage the blood vessels in and towards the kidneys. It is, therefore, an important risk for kidney damage. Stopping smoking ensures that your health immediately jumps. And you notice it: your breathing improves, coughing becomes less, the condition goes up and smelling and tasting goes better.

Moderate drinking
For adult men and women, moderate drinking means on average no more than a standard glass per day. The benefits of drinking alcohol do not outweigh the disadvantages. That is why the advice is not to drink alcohol or at least not more than 1 glass per day. In any case, try to insert a number of alcohol-free days.

Use as little salt as possible
Using minimal salt is very important in preventing kidney damage. Salt can lead to high blood pressure, which is harmful to the kidneys. And salt is also directly harmful to the kidneys, especially if there is kidney damage. Protein loss in the urine - which is detrimental to the kidneys, heart and blood vessels - also decreases due to salt restriction.

TIPS FOR EATING LESS SALT

Eating less salt can delay the worsening of kidney damage. But it can be challenging to reduce salt. Much of the salt that you get is already in the products when you buy them. And you may have to get used to the taste of eating less salt.

These tips help you eat less salt:

- Give yourself time to get used to it
- Choose unprocessed foods
- Do not add salt yourself
- Avoid salty seasonings
- Use herbs, spices, and seasonings such as onion and garlic
- Eat less salty bread meals

- Let someone else cook (sometimes)
- Avoid licorice, liquorice tea, minty Maroc tea, and star mix tea

1. Give yourself time to get used to it

Remember that it takes time to get used to a meal without salt. You have to get rid of the salty taste. This is only possible by consistently not using salt or salty seasonings. In the beginning, less salt food tastes mostly bland, but after a while, you will taste better, and you will find a lot of salt dirty.

2. Choose unprocessed food

Processed foods are products that the manufacturer has processed with salt or other flavorings. These products contain (a lot of) salt. Think of ready-made sauces and soups, and ready-made meals. Avoid processed meat, such as hamburgers, roulade, seasoned minced meat, and sausage. Also, do away with processed fish, such as marinated fresh fish, breaded (frozen) fish, steamed and smoked fish, and canned fish and pickled fish.

Therefore, choose unprocessed food: unprocessed meat, unprocessed chicken, unprocessed fish, and fresh vegetables or frozen vegetables. Season with herbs and spices if necessary.

Ask a butcher to prepare processed meat without salt, such as a low-sodium variant of processed meat like a roulade.

Choose vegetable preserves without added salt: look at the health food store or the supermarket diet

Cook extra portions and store them in the freezer, as an alternative to a salty ready-made meal.

Compare labels

Compare different brands and variants of food. The differences in the amount of salt are large. If you always choose the brand or variant with the least salt, your salt intake will decrease.

3. Do not add salt yourself

Do not add any more salt yourself when cooking. Place the salt pot far away so that you do not grab it automatically.

Also, do not use salt products with other names. Such as:

Celery salt, garlic salt, onion salt, Himalayan salt or Celtic sea salt. These contain just as much salt as common kitchen salt.

Dietary salt, half-salt and mineral salt contain much less sodium than ordinary salt. Potassium is in it instead. If you have a potassium limitation, these products are not a suitable alternative to salt.

Monosodium glutamate (E621): This is a flavor enhancer that contains sodium. It is also known as Chinese salt or Ve-tsin.

4. Avoid salty seasonings
Avoid the use of salty seasonings. For example, Maggi, bouillon cubes, soy sauce, scattering aroma, and soy sauce.

Sodium-limited variant

A sodium-limited version of many flavorings is also available. Ask about it at supermarkets or health food stores. Sodium-limited flavorings often contain potassium. Look at the label. Potassium is also listed as potassium chloride or E508. If you have a potassium restriction, then these sodium-restricted flavorings are not a suitable alternative.

5. Use herbs
Use fresh or dried garden herbs and spices to add flavor to your food.

Avoid ready-to-use spice mixes, ready-to-eat vegetable seeds and spice mixtures such as minced meat. Most of them consist of salt!

Traditional spice mixes such as meat, minced meat, and fish herbs contain salt. But there are also variants without salt for sale: you can often find them in the diet section of the supermarket.

There are many mixed herbs for sale without added salt. They are just in the spice box. Check the label for salt.

6. Eat less salty bread meals
Each slice of bread contains 0.35 grams of salt. Your salt intake decreases if you choose bread without salt. Bread without salt must be ordered from the bakery, or bake yourself.

You also eat less salt if you choose spreads that contain less salt. The siege below contains less salt than 1 slice of regular 48+ Gouda cheese or 1 portion of normally salted meats:

- cheese with less salt (25% or 33% less salt)
- Emmental or Gruyere cheese
- MonChou, cottage cheese
- Mozzarella
- Swiss stray cheese
- slightly salted meats: roast beef, slightly salted smoked meat, fricandeau, turkey breast, chicken breast
- peanut butter
- dairy spread
- sandwich spread, vegetable spread
- fruit: strawberry, apple/pear slices, banana slices
- raw vegetables: radish, cress, cucumber slices
- sweet toppings, such as jam

7. Have someone else cook (sometimes)

Do you not want to or cannot cook without salt? Then there are several other good options. Do not opt for ready-made meals from the supermarket, the butcher or the greengrocer. These contain a lot of salt. Below are some good alternatives.

Open table

Many nursing homes offer residents the option of eating a hot meal for a fee. Diet meals are possible. You must be able to come to the nursing home yourself.

Meals on Wheels

Table-cover-you is a service for the elderly and the long-term sick. You will receive the complete main meals delivered to your home. That can be a hot meal or a cooled meal that you need to heat. Diet meals are possible. Ask about the table at the home care institution in your municipality.

Frozen meals at home

Some organizations deliver frozen meals to order on demand. Diet meals are often also possible.

TIPS FOR EATING LESS SATURATED FAT

People with kidney damage often also have high blood pressure. And an increased amount of fats in the blood, such as cholesterol and triglycerides. High blood pressure and high cholesterol increase the risk of cardiovascular disease.

Eating less saturated fat and more unsaturated fat reduces your risk of cardiovascular disease.

Tips for eating less saturated fat
Choose soft margarine or soft low-fat margarine with at least 50% polyunsaturated fatty acids.

For baking, roasting, and deep-frying, choose soft or liquid fats with a high percentage of unsaturated fat or oil.

Eat fish once a week in particular fatty fish, such as salmon, sardines, and mackerel. Smoked fish contains much more salt than fresh fish.

Limit the use of foods in which saturated fat is hidden, such as cakes, chocolate, and snacks. In some situations, for example, with a poor nutritional status, your dietician may advise you to use these foods temporarily.

Unsaturated fat is better
Fats consist of fatty acids. There are two types: saturated fatty acids and unsaturated fatty acids. Also: saturated fat and unsaturated fat.

Saturated fat raises blood cholesterol. This increases the risk of cardiovascular disease.

Unsaturated fat helps prevent barrels from narrowing. Narrowed and blocked vessels cause cardiovascular disease. Unsaturated fat helps prevent this.

Foods with lots of unsaturated fat are okay:

- all types of oil (including olive oil)
- soft margarine
- liquid cooking fat
- soft low-fat margarine
- nuts
- Fatty fish

Note: some bread spreads are enriched with potassium. These are less suitable if you have a potassium restriction.

Foods with a lot of saturated fat are wrong:

- butter
- margarine in a package
- full-fat cheese
- whole milk products
- whipped cream
- fat meat
- coconut
- chocolate
- pastries and snacks

TIPS AGAINST FOOD INFECTIONS

Good hygiene is always important, even with food that looks good, smells good and tastes great. Because that too can contain bacteria that make you sick.

Tips against food infections
- Only eat cooked foods
- Avoid cross-contamination
- Keep prepared products limited
- Avoid products with listeria bacteria
- Be careful with raw products and soft ice cream
- If you are going on holiday abroad, then additional measures apply. The simpler the circumstances and the warmer the climate, the greater the chance that you will contract a food infection.

1. Only eat cooked foods
Make sure that meat, chicken, and egg are well-cooked before you eat them. The high temperature at which food cooks also kills bacteria.

2. Avoid cross-contamination
During cooking, avoid any contact between raw foods and prepared foods (especially meat, fish and chicken). Otherwise, you contaminate a cooked dish with new bacteria. Take a clean dish towel and kitchen towel daily. Wash it at 60 ° C.

3. Do not store prepared products for too long
You can store prepared products in the fridge for a maximum of 24 hours, provided it is 5 ° C or cooler in the fridge. If the temperature is higher, the food cannot be stored for as long.

4. Avoid products with listeria bacteria
Avoid foods that contain listeria bacteria:

- Raw milk cheese
- Pre-packaged smoked fish
- Raw animal products

5. Avoid raw products and soft ice cream
Avoid products from raw fish and raw meat, such as shrimps and tartar and products with raw egg (such as desserts and meringues) and with soft ice cream.

TIPS AGAINST CONSTIPATION

Constipation is also called slow bowel movements or constipation. It means that pooping is difficult. Blockage can occur as a side effect of certain medicines, such as phosphate binders and iron preparations. But constipation can also be due to a shortage of dietary fiber, a fluid restriction or too little exercise. Constipation is also a side effect of dialysis, in particular, peritoneal dialysis (abdominal flushing). Your lifestyle has a lot of influence on your bowel movements. These tips can help against clogging:

- Eat enough dietary fiber

- Eat regularly
- Go to the toilet if you feel an urge
- Keep moving
- Drink enough (unless you have a fluid restriction)

1. Eat enough dietary fiber
Eat foods rich in dietary fiber. Which are:

- Rye bread, wholemeal bread, and brown bread
- Wholemeal products such as oatmeal, muesli, wheat flakes
- Whole wheat pasta, brown rice,
- Vegetables, raw vegetables, fruit (preferably with peel) and potatoes
- Dried and soaked dried fruits such as plums, apricots, tutti-frutti, and raisins
- Nuts, peanuts
- Legumes, such as brown and white beans, capuchins and lentils

Note: many of these foods are rich in potassium. Keep this in mind if you have a potassium restriction.

2. Eat regularly
Eat regularly. That keeps the intestines moving. It is a personal choice whether you eat something 3 times a day or 5 times. But it is important that your eating rhythm is about the same every day. And at least don't skip your breakfast. Eating at the start of the day stimulates your intestines.

3. Go to the toilet if you feel an urge
Listen to your body. Go to the toilet immediately if you feel an urge. If you stop it, the poo will get hard.

4. Keep moving
Try to move more, as far as possible in your situation. Walking helps better against constipation than cycling or swimming.

5. Drink enough
Do you have no moisture restriction? Then drink 2 to 2.5 liters of fluid per day. Too little moisture can cause dry, hard stools.

STOP SMOKING: 10 PITFALLS AND TIPS.

Pitfall 1. Arrive by weight
The fear of arriving is one of the most important obstacles for people to quit smoking. That fear is partly justified because nicotine speeds up metabolism and by stopping, many smokers gain a few kilos. If this is a tricky issue for you, consider in advance how you can counteract weight gain as much as possible.

Simultaneous dieting and quitting smoking are often discouraged because for most people; it is too much of a good thing. But stopping smoking is another great time to take a closer look at your entire lifestyle. Make a plan in advance in your head how you will handle extra kilos. The one takes a few extra pounds for granted. Another intends to get rid of the kilos in half a year, and another person prevents weight gain by exercising more in advance or paying extra attention to his eating habits.

Pitfall 2. Feeling hungry
Nicotine inhibits appetite and stoppers will get more appetite for food. Stopping smoking also improves your taste and smell, so you can get more hunger. Before you stop, look for recipes that fill well, but that will not make you arrive, for example, meal salads and soups. A soup beforehand will satisfy the worst appetite.

Pitfall 3. Unhealthy snuffers
If you already know that you will fall prey to snails, make sure you have a plan for the difficult moments. Usually, the quiet evenings in front of the tube or with a book are the most difficult. It is almost impossible never to have a blow, but try to limit the amount of snacks or simply do not bring them home. Preferably look for spicy snacks, because you often have enough of these. For example, radishes, cauliflower florets or carrots with garlic dip or tzatziki are very suitable for temporarily reducing the need for a cigarette.

Pitfall 4. Fall into old habits
With smoking addiction, the habit is sometimes more stubborn than

physical addiction. Often not all cigarettes a person smokes a day are needed to meet the physical addiction. Cigarettes can also be lit out of habit, for example, because it is a break or because you are going to drink coffee. For example, if you are used to smoking a cigarette while studying or doing household chores as a moment of rest, try to arrange this break in a different way. Before you stop smoking, try to list those habitual cigarettes and think about how you can capture those moments with other activities.

Pitfall 5. Keep cigarettes and ashtrays
Stopping smoking is hard enough. Don't make it harder on yourself by storing your cigarettes, lighters, and ashtrays. It is better to throw them all away so that you are not reminded of smoking. A partner who also smokes can also hamper your stop-smoking attempt for the same reason, so, therefore, it is advisable for you to quit together. That makes it easier for both of you.

Pitfall 6. Reduce smoking
Some people think it helps to reduce smoking first before you stop. Yet this often does not seem to work! Decreasing alone does not usually improve your health because even small amounts of smoke are already harmful. In addition, people with a disability often go for longer with one cigarette, and they also breathe in the smoke deeper, which ultimately results in almost as many unhealthy substances. It is also very difficult to reduce smoking alone. That is why the tip is to stop smoking cold turkey.

Pitfall 7. Afraid of concentration problems and unrest
Many smokers are afraid of concentration problems and unrest. They are afraid of not being able to work, write or sleep properly. Concentration problems are indeed part of the withdrawal symptoms of smoking. You can avoid these in the first few weeks by using nicotine substitutes such as chewing gum or plasters and gradually reducing them.

Pitfall 8. Use unprepared anti-smoking medication
Anti-smoking medication such as Zyban or Nortrilen is sometimes prescribed by doctors. These antidepressants are used in small doses as an anti-smoking pill. Some smokers benefit, but they are relatively heavy drugs, with the risk of side effects and in the case of Zyban

allergic reactions. So think carefully about what you might use as an aid.

Pitfall 9. Not knowing where to relax
Most smokers cannot escape a tense feeling in the first few weeks, especially those who associate smoking with moments of rest or who relieve stress must find other ways to relax. It is very important to complete this search process before you stop smoking. In the first days of quitting smoking, the stress of quitting is added. And if you're used to relieving stress with a cigarette, you literally don't know where to look. Walking outside, working out, visiting a sauna, a massage, a hot bath, cinema or a good book; make an inventory in advance where you as a brand new non-smoker can get the best relaxation and distraction from and start practicing with it.

Pitfall 10. Not having a good incentive
Before you stop smoking, think about what is an important motivation for you to quit smoking. For some, that is the example for the children, for others, maintaining beautiful skin and for third, healthy lungs. Think of the motivation in the difficult moments, and maybe it can help you to get through the difficult moment.

90+ RECIPES

Ciabatta

Ingredients

- 15 g fresh yeast
- 700 g flour (type 405)
- 5 tbsp milk (1.5% fat)
- 2 tbsp olive oil
- 20 g sea salt
- 200 g fine wheat wholemeal flour
- some flour to work

Preparation

1. Prepare the batter the night before: Dissolve 5 g of yeast in 250-260 ml of lukewarm water in a bowl and let stand for 10 minutes.
2. Sift 350g of flour. Stir with a wooden spoon for 5 minutes until sticky dough is formed.
3. Cover the bowl with cling film and leave for 12 hours at room temperature.
4. Prepare the main dough the next day: Dissolve the remaining yeast in the warm milk and let stand for 10 minutes.
5. Add 250 ml of water (room temperature), olive oil and starter dough and knead with the dough hooks of the hand mixer.
6. Mix salt with remaining flour and fine wholemeal flour and gradually add to the dough, kneading for about 4 minutes.
7. Sprinkle the work surface with flour, put the ciabatta dough on it and knead it vigorously by hand for 2-3 minutes.
8. Lightly oil a bowl. Add ciabatta dough, turn over and cover with cling film. Leave at room temperature for about 1 1/2 hours. The gone ciabatta dough should be very airy, sticky and elastic.
9. Carefully pull with your hand.
10. Generously dust 2 pieces of baking paper with flour and place the loaves of bread on top.

11. Press, in each case a few "dimples" with the fingertips. Dust 2 kitchen towels with flour on one side and cover the ciabatta loaves with them. Let it go for 1 1/2 hours.
12. Place 2 ciabatta loaves with baking paper on a baking tray and sprinkle the oven wall with a little water. Bread in the pre-heated oven at 250 ° C (circulating air: 220 ° C, gas: 4-5) bake for about 20-25 minutes and let cool on an oven rack. Bake the remaining ciabatta loaves in the same way.

Rice with stir-fried chicken fillet and bok choy

Ingredients

- 200 g chicken fillet
- 1 shrub bok choy
- 1 red pepper
- 200 g of rice
- 2 tbsp oil
- 2 tbsp curry
- 1 clove of garlic, chopped
- ½ red pepper, chopped without seeds
- 1 cup of crème Fraiche

Preparation

1. Cut the chicken into cubes. Clean the bok choy and cut the stems and leaves into strips of approximately 2 centimeters. Clean the bell pepper and cut it into small strips.
2. Prepare the rice according to the instructions on the package. In the meantime, heat the oil in a wok (or frying pan) and stir-fry the chicken until brown, then fry the garlic and chili.
3. Sprinkle the chicken with the curry and stir in the bok choy and bell pepper. Stir fry the whole for another 5 minutes.
4. Drain the rice well.
5. Stir the crème fraîche into the meat and vegetable mixture and stir-fry until everything is thoroughly hot.
6. Season the dish with pepper.

Amaranth muesli bars

Ingredients

- 50 g flaked almonds
- 40 g sunflower seeds
- 25 g peanut kernel (unsalted)
- 50 g 5-grain cereal flakes
- 30 g puffamaranth
- 1 tsp cinnamon
- 25 g sultanas
- 1 pinch salt
- 75 g butter
- 50 g cane sugar
- 4 tbsp liquid honey

Preparation

1. Put almond flakes, sunflower seeds, peanut kernels, cereal flakes, amaranth and dates in a bowl. Add cinnamon, sultanas, and salt and mix well.
2. Melt the butter in a saucepan over low heat. Add sugar and honey and bring to a boil over medium heat with constant stirring.
3. Add hot sugar mixture to the remaining ingredients and mix thoroughly with a wooden spoon. Lay out a springform pan (24 cm) with baking paper and add the mixture.
4. Press firmly and bake in a pre-heated oven at 180 ° C (circulating air: not recommended, gas: stage 2-3) for about 25 minutes. Allow cooling completely, release from the mold and cut into triangles.

Red Currant Jelly

Ingredients

- 1800 g red currants
- 500 g gelling sugar made from whole cane sugar 3: 1

- 12 coffee beans

Preparation

1. Wash currants and drain well.
2. Using a fork, brush the berries off the stems.
3. Place the berries in a large saucepan and add 150 ml of water. Cover the berries and bring them to a boil for about 30 minutes, stirring occasionally.
4. Lay out a fine sieve with a kitchen towel and hang over a pot. Pour berries and juice into the strainer and drain thoroughly for 5-6 hours. Meanwhile, wash 4 screw jars (400 ml each) and rinse the appropriate lid with boiling water and drain headfirst on a kitchen towel.
5. Measure 1.2 l of juice. Put in a saucepan with gelling sugar and mix.
6. Place the coffee beans in a kitchen towel, seal with kitchen yarn and add to the pot with the juice.
7. Bring the juice to a boil while stirring constantly.
8. When boiling, boil off with a foam trowel, and boil the juice bubbly for 4 minutes.
9. Remove the coffee bean bag.
10. Fill the prepared glasses with hot liquid and close with the lids. Leave for about 5 minutes, then stand upright again.

Raspberry Jelly with Mint

Ingredients

- 2 kg raspberries
- 4 stems mint
- 500 g gelierzucker 3: 1

Preparation

1. Read raspberries, rinse carefully in a sieve and drain well.

2. Place the berries in a large saucepan and add 150 ml of water. Cover the berries and bring to a boil. Let them simmer for about 30 minutes, stirring occasionally.
3. Lay out a fine sieve with a kitchen towel and hang over a pot. Strain berries and juice and drain thoroughly for 5-6 hours. Meanwhile, 4 screw jars (400 ml each) and rinse the appropriate lid with boiling water and drain headfirst on a kitchen towel.
4. Wash mint and shake dry. Pluck leaves.
5. Measure 1.2 l of juice. Put the gelling sugar in a saucepan and stir.
6. Bring the juice to a boil while stirring constantly.
7. When boiling boil off foam with a skimmer and boil the juice while stirring bubbly for 4 minutes.
8. Add mint and cook for another 30 seconds.
9. Fill the prepared glasses with hot liquid and cover with lids. Leave for about 5 minutes.

Blackberry and Elderberry Jelly

Ingredients

- 1400 g blackberry
- 600 g elderberries
- 500 g gelierzucker 3: 1
- ½ lemon

Preparation

1. Wash the blackberries and drain well.
2. Rinse elderberries, drain well and pluck from the stems.
3. Put all the berries in a saucepan and add 150 ml of water.
4. Cover slowly and bring to a boil. Simmer covered for about 30 minutes, stirring gently from time to time.
5. Lay out a fine sieve with a kitchen towel and hang over a pot. Put the berries in the sieve and drain thoroughly for about 5-6 hours. In the meantime, rinse 3 screw jars (400 ml each) with matching lids with boiling water and drain upside down on a kitchen towel.
6. Measure a total of 1.2 l from the drained berry juice. Put the gelling sugar in the pot and bring to a boil, stirring constantly.

7. When cooking, remove the rising foam with a skimmer and let the juice boil for 4-6 minutes. Squeeze out the lemon. Stir 2 tablespoons of lemon juice under the jelly and cook for another 30 seconds.
8. Hot fill the liquid into the prepared glasses and close immediately. Leave for about 5 minutes, then stand upright again.

Papaya and orange jam

Ingredients

- 1000 g papaya (2 papayas)
- 500 g oranges (3 oranges)
- 500 g gelierzucker 3: 1

Preparation

1. Peel papayas, cut in half and remove the seeds.
2. Cut the pulp into small cubes.
3. Peel oranges so thick that all white skin is removed.
4. Remove the pulp from the skins and add to the papaya cubes. Squeeze the skins thoroughly and mix the juice with the fruit. All together should weigh about 1.3 kg.
5. Add the jelly sugar, mix everything thoroughly and leave for about 2 hours. In the meantime, rinse 4 screw jars (400 ml each) with matching lids with boiling water and drain upside down on a kitchen towel.
6. Put the papaya and orange mix in a saucepan, bring to a boil while stirring and then boil for 4 minutes while stirring.
7. Fill the prepared glasses with hot liquid and cover with lids. Leave for about 5 minutes, then stand upright again.

Carrot drink

Ingredients

- 2 small cloves of garlic

- 800 g bunch of carrots
- 1 bunch smooth parsley
- ½ lemon
- 1 tsp rapeseed oil

Preparation

1. Peel garlic cloves.
2. Thoroughly wash carrots and cut off the ends.
3. Wash the parsley and shake dry. Squeeze lemon half off.
4. Juice garlic and 6 carrots in the juicer.
5. Add parsley and remaining carrots to the juicer and juice.
6. Mix carrot drink with about 2 tablespoons of lemon juice and the rapeseed oil and enjoy immediately.

Spicy Apple and Pineapple Juice

Ingredients

- 600 g apples (3 apples)
- ¼ pineapple (about 250 g of pulp)
- 25 g ginger root (1 piece)
- ½ lime

Preparation

1. Wash apples and cut small.
2. Peel the pineapple, remove the hard core and cut the pulp into large pieces.
3. Peel ginger and dice roughly. Squeeze out the lime.
4. Add apples, pineapple, and ginger to a juicer and juice. Season with lime juice and enjoy as quickly as possible.

Green fruit packets

Ingredients

- 200 g green seedless grapes
- 2 kiwis
- 300 g green-colored pears (2 green-colored pears)
- 300 g small melon (e.g. galia, 0.5 small melons)
- 8 g ginger (1 piece)
- 1 cinnamon stick
- 4 cardamom pods
- 4 tbsp maple syrup

Preparation

1. Wash the grapes, drain in a colander, pluck from the stems and cut in half.
2. Peel and slice the kiwis.
3. Wash pears, quarter, core and cut into slices.
4. Core melon with a teaspoon, cut into slices and peel.
5. Ginger peel and finely chop. Break the cinnamon stick into 4 small pieces.
6. From the baking paper cut 4 pieces of about 35x25 cm each.
7. Divide grapes, kiwi, pears and melon and ginger into 4 portions and put 1 serving in the middle of 1 piece of baking paper.
8. Add 1 piece of cinnamon stick and 1 cardamom pod and dribble 1 tbsp of maple syrup.
9. Fold the baking paper into small packets and close.
10. Cook in a preheated oven at 180 ° C (circulating air: 160 ° C, gas: stage 2-3) for about 15-20 minutes. Put on a plate, open slightly and serve.

Strawberry papaya drink

Ingredients

- 2 stems mint
- 250 g strawberries

- 2 kiwis
- 400 g papaya (1 papaya)

Preparation

1. Wash the mint, shake dry, peel off the leaves and set aside.
2. Wash strawberries carefully, drain on kitchen paper, clean, chop and place in a tall container. Puree with a hand blender and strain into 2 glasses.
3. Peel kiwis, halve, dice and place in a tall container. Purée with the hand blender and place gently with a spoon on the strawberry puree.
4. Halve the papaya and remove the seeds with a spoon. Remove the pulp from the skin, chop it roughly and puree with the hand blender. Carefully pour into jars, garnish with mint and serve immediately.

Orange Bulgur

Ingredients

- 100 g bulgur
- 300 g large organic orange (250-1 large organic orange)
- ½ tl rapeseed oil
- 125 g small apples (1 small apple)
- 125 g small pears (1 small pear)
- 100 g grapes
- 1 fresh fig
- 125 g small bananas (1 small banana)
- ½ lime
- 2 tsp maple syrup

Preparation

1. Put bulgur in a bowl. Brew with 100 ml of boiling water and allow to swell for about 5 minutes.

2. Meanwhile, wash orange, rub dry and finely rub the skin. Halve orange, squeeze out and measure 120 ml of juice. Mix the juice, peel and rape oil with a fork under the swollen bulgur.
3. Wash the apple, pear, grapes, and fig and pat dry. Quarter a pear and apple. Cut the grapes in half and remove them if necessary, peel the banana. Cut all fruits into bite-sized pieces.
4. Squeeze half the lime and stir the juice in a small bowl with the maple syrup. Pour over the fruits, mix everything and leave to soak for 8-10 minutes. Serve with the orange bulgur and serve.

Artichoke cream on corn waffles

Ingredients

- 120 g small tomatoes (3 small tomatoes)
- 220 g Artichoke bottoms (can, drained weight)
- 5 g ground almonds (1 tsp)

    - salt
    - pepper

- 4 stems basil
- 2 corn waffle

Preparation

1. Wash the tomatoes, cut out the stems into a wedge shape.
2. 2 quarters tomatoes; remove seeds and cut into 5 mm cubes.
3. Drain 3 artichoke bottoms, then cut into 1 cm pieces. Puree the half in a tall container with a hand blender.
4. Mix the artichoke puree with artichoke pieces, diced tomatoes and ground almonds. Season with salt, pepper and leave for 10 minutes.
5. Rinse the basil, shake dry and peel off the leaves. Put some aside for garnish, cut the rest into fine strips.
6. Stir under the artichoke cream, season with salt and pepper again and spread on the corn waffles. Garnish with basil leaves and serve.

Oat and pine nut crunchies

Ingredients

- 75 g pine nuts (or almonds)
- 250 g hearty oatmeal
- 2 tsp cinnamon
- 1 pinch salt
- 50 ml honey
- 50 ml maple syrup
- 2 tbsp rapeseed oil
- 50 g dried cherries

Preparation

1. Chop pine nuts, place in a bowl with the oatmeal. Add cinnamon and salt and mix everything.
2. Mix the honey, maple syrup and oil in a saucepan and bring to the boil while stirring.
3. Carefully lift with a wooden spoon under the mixture of flakes.
4. Lay out a baking sheet with baking paper and spread the mixture of flakes on it.
5. Bake in a preheated oven at 125 ° C (circulating air: 110 ° C, gas: stage 1-2) for approx. 1 1/4 hours, turning carefully 2 to 3 times.
6. Remove from the oven and allow to cool completely. Then mix the crunchies with the dried cherries. Fill in an airtight sealable glass; That's how the crunchies last for about 3 weeks. Remove by the portion.

Mango and raspberry cocktail

Ingredients

- 350 g ripe mango (1 ripe mango)
- 200 g pink grapefruit (1 pink grapefruit)
- 2 stems mint

- 150 g raspberries
- mineral water at will
- also: ice cubes

Preparation

1. Wash the mango and peel with a peeler. Slice the pulp from the stone and dice it.
2. Halve the grapefruit and squeeze it out.
3. Wash mint, shake dry, peel off leaves and cut into thin strips.
4. If necessary, gently rinse the raspberries, drain, and place with the mango cubes and grapefruit juice in a tall container. Puree with a hand blender and mix until foamy. Add ice cubes to glasses, fill with mineral water as desired and garnish with mint strips.

Melons and spinach juice

Ingredients

- 350 g small honeydew melon (0.5 small honeydew melons)
- 250 g young tender spinach leaves
- 1 piece cinnamon stick (about 1 cm)
- nutmeg
- also: ice cubes

Preparation

1. Core the melon with a teaspoon. First cut the melon into slices, then cut the flesh from the shell and chop it roughly.
2. Clean the spinach and wash thoroughly in a bowl of water. Repeat the water several times until it stays clear.
3. Scrape thin strips off the cinnamon stick with a small sharp knife.
4. Express the spinach lightly; move a small leaflet and a small stalk for the garnish. Juice the rest with the melon in a juicer and pour ice cubes into a glass. Garnish with some nutmeg, garnish with cinnamon and possibly the spinach and enjoy immediately.

Baguette

Ingredients

- 250 g wheat flour type 550
- 225 g whole-wheat flour
- 15 g fresh yeast
- 12 g salt (2 tsp)
- 1 tbsp rapeseed oil

Preparation

1. On the eve of the pre-dough, put 125 g wheat flour and 75 g wheat wholegrain flour in a bowl. Break in 10 g of yeast and add 250 ml of lukewarm water.
2. Knead with the dough hook of the hand mixer for 1 minute. Cover well with cling film and let it rest for at least 12 hours at room temperature.
3. The next day, add the remaining flour and remaining whole wheat flour with salt in a bowl and in the middle of a depression. The remaining yeast crumbles in. Add 125 ml of lukewarm water and let rest for 10 minutes.
4. Add the dough to the other ingredients in the bowl and knead with the kneading hook of the hand mixer for 4 minutes.
5. Place the dough on a floured surface and knead for another 10 minutes by hand, possibly adding some flour until the dough no longer sticks to the hands.
6. Add oil to a bowl and turn the dough ball in it to wet the surface. Cover with cling film and leave at room temperature for 1 1/2 hours until the volume has doubled.
7. Lightly knead the dough together and form into an elongated loaf. Let it go for another 60 minutes.
8. Place the piece of dough on the floured work surface and quarter.
9. Bring the pieces of dough together by pressing lightly and rolling them in baguette sticks (about 25 cm in length).
10. Place the baguette pieces of dough on a baking tray covered with baking paper and leave to stand covered with a floured kitchen towel for 40 minutes.

11. Carve the baguettes diagonally several times with a very sharp knife. Bake in a preheated oven at 220 ° C (circulating air 200 ° C, gas: stage 3-4) on the second rail from below for 30-35 minutes.
12. Allow baguettes to cool on the oven rack before serving.

Avocado toast with cilantro

Ingredients

- 4 lime
- 300 ml tomato juice
- worcester sauce
- tabasco
- salt
- black pepper
- 1 small red onion
- ½ lemon
- 2 tbsp olive oil
- 1 avocado
- 2 slices sourdough crusty bread
- a little coriander

Preparation

1. Squeeze out limes the day before, mix 8 tablespoons of lime juice with 4 tablespoons of water and freeze to cubes in the ice cube maker.
2. Mix tomato juice with Worcester sauce, Tabasco, a little salt and pepper. Cover with cold cover.
3. Peel the onion and chop finely. Squeeze out the lemon. Mix 1 tbsp lemon juice with salt, pepper, and onion cubes. Embezzle olive oil.
4. Halve the avocado, remove the stone. Using a spoon, lift the avocado meat from its shells and cut into slices
5. Add avocado to the onions, mix gently and let stand for 15 minutes.

6. Toast the bread in the toaster or under the hot oven grill from both sides golden yellow. Wash cilantro, shake dry and peel off the leaves.
7. Put the avocado on the slices of bread and sprinkle with cilantro.
8. Put 2 lime ice cubes into 2 small glasses and pour over the tomato juice. For decoration, slightly moisten the edges of the glasses and dip in salt.

Apple and celery spread

Ingredients

- 2 msp. curry powder
- 100 g buttermilk cream cheese (0.2% fat)
- 1 pole celery
- 150 g small apples (1 small apple)
- salt
- pepper

Preparation

1. Mix curry powder with 2 tablespoons of warm water. Add cream cheese and stir until creamy.
2. Wash celery, remove and clean if necessary. Finely chop the green, finely chop the celery. Put 1 tbsp celery cube aside.
3. Wash the apple, rub dry, quarter and remove the core. Finely dice the apple.
4. Mix curry cream cheese with apples, celery, and celery green. If the mass is too firm, add 1-2 tablespoons of water and stir until creamy. Season the spread with salt and pepper and sprinkle with remaining celery cubes.

Ayurveda muesli

Ingredients

- 20 g ginger (1 piece)
- 120 g fine 5-grain cereal mixture or oatmeal
- 2 tsp maple syrup
- 200 g sour apples (1 sour apple)
- 150 g pears (1 pear)
- 1 tsp ghee
- cinnamon

Preparation

1. Peel ginger and finely grate.
2. Put the cereal, ginger and 500 ml of water in a saucepan, bring to the boil and simmer for 3-5 minutes over low heat while stirring. Sweeten with maple syrup.
3. Wash apple and pear, drizzle dry. Quarter the fruits, core them and cut into slices.
4. Heat ghee in another pot. Add apple and pear slices and simmer for 2-3 minutes over low heat. Season with cinnamon.
5. Grain porridge and fruit compote in glasses layers.

Pineapple Amaranth bars

Ingredients

- 100 g dried pineapple
- 2 tbsp butter
- 100 g liquid honey
- 2 tbsp whole cane sugar
- ½ lime
- 100 g oatmeal
- 50 g amaranth pops
- 4 tbsp chopped almonds

Preparation

1. Cut pineapple into small cubes.
2. Bring butter, honey, and sugar to a boil.
3. Squeeze out the lime.
4. Mix 1 tbsp lime juice, oatmeal, amaranth, almonds and pineapple cube with the sweet butter.
5. Spread the mixture with a damp rubber spatula approx. 2 cm thick on a baking tray lined with baking paper and bake in the preheated oven at 150 ° C (circulating air 130 ° C, gas: 1-2) on the middle rail for 15-18 minutes.
6. Cut into bars while still warm and let cool on a work board. Store in tightly closed boxes.

Juicy wheat bread

Ingredients

- 430 g flour
- ¼ tl dry yeast
- 2 tsp sea salt
- maize semolina

Preparation

1. Mix the flour in a bowl with yeast and salt. Slowly add 340 ml of lukewarm water while stirring.
2. Cover the bowl with cling film. Let the dough rise at room temperature for 24 hours.
3. For processing, dust the work surface well with flour. Carefully remove the dough from the bowl and place on the work surface.
4. Flatten gently with your hands and fold from two sides to the middle.
5. From the other sides also fold to the middle.
6. Sprinkle a large kitchen towel generously with cornstarch and place the dough down with the seam.
7. Sprinkle the dough surface with semolina and fold the kitchen towel over the dough or use a second cloth to cover. Let the dough again for about 2 hours, until the volume has doubled. Preheat the

oven to 250 ° C (circulating air: 220 ° C, gas: level 4) and heat a heavy pot (cast iron or enamel) in it for about 30 minutes.
8. Place the bread dough on a piece of baking paper and place it carefully in the hot pot. Put the lid on and bake the bread for 5 minutes. Then reduce the temperature to 200 ° C (circulating air 180 ° C, gas: level 3) and bake for another 25 minutes. Now remove the lid and continue baking the bread for another 25-30 minutes. Take the wheat bread and let it cool down completely on an oven rack.

Papaya Orange Smoothie

Ingredients

- 200 g small papaya (1 small papaya)
- 8th juice oranges
- 100 g raspberries (frozen)
- 1 stalk lemon balm (at will)

1. Preparation
2. Peel and halve the papaya and remove the seeds with a spoon.
3. Cut the pulp into large pieces.
4. Squeeze oranges.
5. Add papaya and orange juice to the blender. Add the raspberries frozen directly from the pack. Mix everything to a smooth, liquid puree. Garnish as desired with lemon balm leaves and serve immediately.

Sweet rice porridge

Ingredients

- 7½ dl of milk
- 250 g of rice
- 250 g of sugar
- grated zest of 1 lemon
- 1 cinnamon stick

- cinnamon powder
- 3 egg yolks

Preparation

1. Bring the milk to the boil.
2. Add the rice, sugar, lemon zest and cinnamon stick when the milk is boiling.
3. Remove the pan from the heat when the rice is cooked. Remove the cinnamon stick.
4. Allow to cool for 5 minutes.
5. Beat the egg yolks and add them to the rice mixture.
6. Mix everything well together.
7. Place the pan over medium heat and keep it on the boil for 5 to 10 minutes. Be careful that it doesn't matter.
8. Let cool well. Serve cold with some cinnamon powder.

Roast beef roast

Ingredients

- 4 tbsp olive oil
- ¼ tsp dried basil
- ¼ tsp dragon
- pepper
- 250 g roast beef in one piece
- ½ tomato
- ½ root
- ½ medium onion
- ½ celery stick
- 1 clove of garlic
- olive oil for frying
- ¼ glass of red wine
1. Preparation
2. Mix the 4 tbsp olive oil with the basil, tarragon, and pepper until smooth.

3. Rub the roast beef with this and let it marinate overnight in the fridge.
4. Preheat the oven to 160 - 170 degrees on the day of preparation.
5. Finely chop the tomato, carrot, onion and celery sticks.
6. Heat some olive oil in a frying pan and fry the meat alternately brown in about 3 minutes per side.
7. Grease a baking dish and put the meat in it.
8. Add the tomato mixture and the garlic and pour in the wine and some water.
9. Bake the meat in the oven. In general, the baking time per 500 grams is 30 minutes for medium and 45 minutes for baking. Occasionally pour some of the baking water over the meat.
10. At the end of the cooking time, remove the meat from the baking dish.
11. Puree the vegetables and the cooking liquid and let it reduce by half.
12. Slice the meat and add the sauce.

Gazpacho

Ingredients

- 2 slices of white bread
- 250 g of tomatoes
- ½ bell pepper (green or red)
- ½ cucumber
- ¼ onion
- ½ clove of garlic
- 1 tbsp olive oil
- vinegar to taste

Preparation

1. Cut the crusts off the bread. The crusts are not used. Crumble the rest of the bread.
2. Peel the tomatoes, remove the seeds and cut the rest into small pieces.

3. Mix the tomatoes and the breadcrumbs with a mixer until a smooth cream appears.
4. Cut the bell pepper and cucumber into small pieces and chop the onion finely.
5. Clean the garlic and crush it.
6. Add everything to the tomato mix.
7. Add a little water and mix everything into a smooth thick soup.
8. Add oil and vinegar.
9. Allow the soup to cool well in 2 to 3 hours in the refrigerator.

Couscous salad

Ingredients

- 125 g couscous
- 4 spring onions
- 1 red pepper
- ½ zucchini
- 50 g peas (frozen)
- 1 lemon
- 50 g fresh parsley
- 1 tsp fresh mint
- 1 tbsp fresh coriander
- 5 tbsp olive oil
- pepper

Preparation

1. Prepare the couscous according to the instructions on the package.
2. Allow the couscous to cool.
3. Meanwhile, wash the spring onions and cut into rings.
4. Also, clean the bell pepper and zucchini and cut into small cubes.
5. Cook the peas briefly and drain them.
6. Rinse the green peas with cold water and drain them.
7. Finely chop the fresh herbs.
8. Squeeze the lemon over a large bowl and season with pepper.

9. Add the couscous and all other ingredients and mix everything well.

Niçoise pasta salad

Ingredients

- 150 g (whole grain) pasta: shells or pipe rigate
- 75 g green beans (or haricots verts)
- 2 eggs
- 150 g cherry tomatoes
- 100 g cucumber
- 3 black olives
- 150 g canned tuna steak (on water)
- 1 tsp Dyon mustard
- 2 tbsp olive oil
- 1 tbsp wine vinegar
- pepper

Preparation

1. Cook the pasta according to the instructions on the package and rinse with cold water.
2. Remove the dots from the green beans and cook them for approx. 10 minutes.
3. Bring water to the boil, boil the eggs for 7 minutes and rinse with cold water. Peel the eggs and cut into quarters.
4. Cut the cherry tomatoes in half and first cut the cucumber into strips and then into pieces.
5. Cut the olives into thin rings.
6. Beat a dressing of mustard, olive oil, and vinegar.
7. Mix the pasta, tomatoes, cucumber pieces and the dressing together in a salad bowl.
8. Divide the tuna steak and green beans over the pasta, sprinkle with tuna rings, put the egg slices on top.
9. Sprinkle with freshly ground pepper as desired.

Pasta with avocado pesto and broccoli

Ingredients

- 200 g (whole grain) pasta
- 300 g broccoli florets
- 1 lemon, waxed
- 1 avocado
- 1 large hand fresh basil (approx. 20 g)
- 2 cloves of garlic
- 25 g pine nuts
- 30 g grated Parmesan cheese
- freshly ground pepper
- 2 tbsp olive oil
- Requirements: food processor or hand blender

1. Preparation
2. Cook the pasta according to the instructions on the package. When draining the pasta, save ¼ cup of water for the pesto.
3. Cook the broccoli florets in about 8 minutes until done.
4. Grate half a zest of the lemon and squeeze the fruit. Cut the avocado in half, remove the kernel and cut into strips. Spoon the strips out of the peel.
5. In a food processor, add the basil, garlic, pine nuts, Parmesan cheese, zest of half lemon, juice of a whole lemon and some freshly ground pepper. Mix everything well and gradually add the olive oil while mixing and mix until smooth. Then add the avocado and the remaining pasta water. Mix everything well again.
6. Add the sauce to the cooked pasta and stir well so that it is completely covered with the sauce. Finally, add the broccoli to the pasta and serve.

Fish package with cod

Ingredients

- 400 g of rice
- 4 sheets of aluminum foil
- dash of oil
- dash of coconut milk
- 400 g zucchini
- 400 g fennel
- 4 pieces of cod of approximately 100 grams
- 2 tbsp dill
- 2 lemons
- black pepper or 4-season pepper

Preparation

Heat the oven to 180 ° C.

1. Cook the rice according to the instructions on the package.
2. Cut the zucchini into cubes and the fennel into slices.
3. Put the aluminum foil down and spread the rice over it with some oil and coconut milk. Place the zucchini and fennel on top and then place the cod on the rice and vegetables. Divide the dill over the packages.
4. Squeeze one of the lemons and cut the other into segments. Divide the juice and the segments over the packages. Add pepper to taste.
5. Fold the packages tightly. (No steam may escape.)
6. Place the packets in the oven for 20-25 minutes (depending on the thickness of the fish).

Spaghetti with kale and meatballs

Ingredients

- 350 g half-to-half minced meat
- 300 g sliced kale
- 1 rusk

- 1 tbsp dried oregano
- 2 tsp Jonnie Boer Picadillo (spice mix)
- 250 g mushrooms in pieces
- 2 tbsp liquid fry & roast
- freshly ground pepper
- 1 onion, chopped
- 300 g (whole grain) spaghetti
- 2 cloves of garlic, chopped
- piece of Parmesan cheese
- 4 sun-dried tomatoes (in oil) in pieces

Preparation

1. Put the minced meat in a bowl, crumble the rusk above it and sprinkle with the spice mix. Knead well together and make small meatballs.
2. Heat the frying pan in a frying pan with a small dash of oil (from the sun-dried tomatoes). Bake the meatballs brown, add a splash of water and cook for about 10 minutes with the lid on the pan. Keep warm with a lid on the pan.
3. Bring a pan of water to the boil for the spaghetti (add the spaghetti later).
4. Heat 2 tablespoons of oil in a wok and fry the onion until it is glassy, then add the garlic and the tomato pieces and fry for 1 minute. Add the kale and stir until it has shrunk. Add a tablespoon of boiling water. Put a lid on the pan and let it simmer for 20 minutes. Add the oregano after 15 minutes.
5. In another frying pan, heat a tablespoon of oil and add the mushrooms with freshly ground pepper. Allow the moisture to evaporate and then bake until golden brown, stirring.
6. Cook the spaghetti at the same time.
7. Spoon the spaghetti and mushrooms into the wok and mix in the kale.
8. Serve the spaghetti with the minced meatballs. Grate some Parmesan cheese on the plate.

Couscous with pumpkin and chickpeas

Ingredients

- 1 bottle squash
- 1 tbsp liquid frying fat
- 2 tbsp honey
- 200 g couscous
- 1 orange, waxed
- 400 g canned chickpeas
- 4 tbsp olive oil
- 2 tsp ras el hanout (for example from Jonnie de Boer or Pure Spices from firm Verstegen)
- 75 g raisins

1. Preparation
2. Preheat the oven to 200 ° C.
3. Wash the pumpkin and halve the length. Remove the seeds and stringy inside with a spoon. Leave the skin on. Cut both halves into 1 cm cubes.
4. Grease the baking sheet with liquid baking & roasting (or use baking paper).
5. Mix the pumpkin with the honey and spread on the greased baking sheet.
6. Bake the pumpkin in the oven for about 20 minutes until the pumpkin is cooked. Scoop halfway through once.
7. Meanwhile, prepare the couscous according to the instructions on the package.
8. Grate the orange zest of the orange and squeeze the fruit.
9. Drain the chickpeas in a colander and rinse with cold running water.
10. Mix the couscous with orange zest and juice, chickpeas, olive oil, ras el hanout, and raisins.
11. Divide the pumpkin on the couscous.

Melons and spinach juice

Ingredients

- 350 g small honeydew melon (0.5 small honeydew melons)
- 250 g young tender spinach leaves
- 1 piece cinnamon stick (about 1 cm)
- nutmeg
- also: ice cubes

Preparation

1. Core the melon with a teaspoon. First cut the melon into slices, then cut the flesh from the shell and chop it roughly.
2. Clean the spinach and wash thoroughly in a bowl of water. Repeat the water several times until it stays clear.
3. Scrape thin strips off the cinnamon stick with a small sharp knife.
4. Express the spinach lightly; move a small leaflet and a small stalk for the garnish. Juice the rest with the melon in a juicer and pour ice cubes into a glass. Garnish with some nutmeg, garnish with cinnamon and possibly the spinach and enjoy immediately.

Exotic smoothie

Ingredients

- 300 g small ripe mango (1 small ripe mango)
- 150 g small ripe bananas (1 small ripe banana)
- 1 lime
- 3 stems lemon balm
- 200 ml whey
- also: ice cubes

Preparation

1. Wash, dry and peel the mango. Slice the flesh from the stone and put aside 2 thin slices. Dice remaining pulp.

2. Peel the banana and crush it on a plate. Squeeze out the lime and drizzle the juice over the banana.
3. Rinse lemon balm, shake dry, peel off leaves and set aside.
4. Put remaining melissa leaves with mango, banana, and whey in a tall container and puree with the hand blender. Sprinkle with ice cubes in 2 glasses, garnish with mango slices and lemon balm.

Papaya Orange Smoothie

Ingredients

- 200 g small papaya (1 small papaya)
- 8th juice oranges
- 100 g raspberries (frozen)
- 1 stalk lemon balm (at will)

Preparation

1. Peel and halve the papaya and remove the seeds with a spoon.
2. Cut the pulp into large pieces.
3. Squeeze oranges.
4. Add papaya and orange juice to the blender. Add the raspberries frozen directly from the pack. Mix everything to a smooth, liquid puree. Garnish as desired with lemon balm leaves and serve immediately.

Pomegranate Juice

Ingredients

- 4 pomegranates
- 25 g ginger (1 piece)
- ½ lemon
- 2 tbsp honey

Preparation

1. Halve the pomegranates and squeeze like oranges on a citrus press.
2. Peel ginger and finely grate.
3. Squeeze out the lemon, mix with ginger and add to the pomegranate juice.
4. Finally, stir the honey under the pomegranate juice. Serve immediately.

Apple cherry cocktail

Ingredients

- 200 g red apples (1 red apple)
- 200 g celery (2 sticks)
- 200 g sour cherries (pitted, frozen)

Preparation

1. Wash, dry, halve and dice the apple.
2. Wash the celery stalks, clean them, remove them if necessary and cut into pieces.
3. Wash the celery green and shake dry.
4. Juice the apple and celery with about 2/3 of the celery green juice in a juicer.
5. Add chilled cherries to the juice and puree with a hand blender. Pour into a glass and garnish with the remaining celery green.

Apple avocado smoothie

Ingredients

- ½ little lemon
- 75 g ripe avocado (0.5 ripe avocados)
- 80 g ripe kiwi (1 ripe kiwi)
- 50 ml naturally cloudy apple juice
- 100 ml mineral water (ice cold)
- also: ice cubes

Preparation

1. Squeeze lemon half and put the juice in a tall container. Remove the stone from the avocado half.
2. Remove the pulp from the avocado with a teaspoon and add immediately to the lemon juice in the jar.
3. Peel kiwi, cut 2 slices and set aside. Dice the rest of the kiwi and add the apple juice to the avocado. Puree everything with a hand blender and pour ice cubes into a large glass. Fill with mineral water and garnish with the kiwi slices.

Ginger lemon orange

Ingredients

- 125 g ginger (1 piece)
- 100 g cane sugar
- 2 limes (1 of them in organic quality)
- 2 oranges (1 of them in organic quality)
- liquid sweetener at will
- cold mineral water at will
- 4 stems mint
- also: ice cubes

Preparation

1. Peel ginger and rub on a fine grater.
2. Boil 1.25 l water and sugar, add the grated ginger and cook for 1 minute. Wash the organic lime and orange, rub dry and peel the peel thinly with a peeler.
3. Put the citrus peel in a decanter, pour over the hot liquid. Allow to cool at room temperature.
4. Halve all fruits and squeeze out. Pour citrus juice into the carafe. Cover Ginger Beer with a kitchen towel and let it rest in a cool, dark place for 24 hours.
5. Pour Ginger Beer the next day through a fine sieve, possibly with some sweet sweetener. Add ice cubes, and fill to taste with a little

mineral water. Wash mint, shake dry and peel off the leaves. Serve ginger beer with lime and orange slices and some mint garnish.

Green carrot mix

Ingredients

- 300 g carrots (2 carrots)
- 2 frets smooth parsley
- 1 pinch cane sugar
- ½ tl pumpkin seed oil
- also: ice cubes

Preparation

1. Wash the carrots, clean them and peel off a few very thin strips of carrot with a peeler. Cut the rest and the 2nd carrot into pieces.
2. Wash the parsley well, shake it dry and chop it roughly with a large knife.
3. Add carrots with parsley, 1 pinch of sugar, oil and the ice cubes in a blender. Slightly foamy, pour into a glass and garnish with carrot strips. Enjoy immediately.

Apple Vegetable Juice

Ingredients

- 300 g carrots (3 carrots)
- 400 g apples (2 apples)
- 250 g tubers red beetroot (2 tubers beetroot)
- ½ lemon
- 1 tsp rapeseed oil

Preparation

1. Carrot thoroughly and cut small. Wash apples, quarter and possibly core.

2. Thoroughly wash the beetroot, peel it with a peeler as desired, or chop it roughly with the peel, possibly working with gloves because of the color.
3. Juice carrots, apples, and beets with a mechanical juicer.
4. Squeeze out the lemon and measure 2 tablespoons of juice. Stir with the rapeseed oil under the apple and vegetable juice and serve immediately.

Pears and kiwi fruit smoothie

Ingredients

- 140 g ripe kiwi (2 ripe kiwis)
- 200 g small ripe pears (2 small ripe pears)
- 1 small lime
- also: ice cubes

Preparation

1. Peel and dice the kiwis.
2. Wash the pears, pat dry, quarter, core and also dice.
3. Rinse the lime, rub dry and peel the peel with a julienne burger in thin strips (julienne).
4. Squeeze out the lime. Puree the kiwi and pears with ice cubes in a blender (or with a hand blender in a tall container). Mix with lime juice, garnish with lime julienne and enjoy immediately.

Aroma water with rosemary

Ingredients

- 1/2 orange, unsprayed
- 1 sprig of rosemary
- 1 liter of mineral water, cooled

Preparation

Rub the sprig of rosemary between your fingers so that it can deliver its aroma better. Cut the orange into thin slices. Put both in a container and fill with mineral water. Let it rest for 30 minutes.

Ginger Tea

Ingredients

- 1-liter red fruit tea
- 1 piece of fresh ginger
- 50g honey
- 2 tablespoons of lemon juice

Preparation

Peel and slice the ginger. Add lemon juice and honey to the hot tea and let it steep for 10 min. To taste, sweeten with candy.

Latte macchiato with white chocolate

Ingredients

- 25 g white chocolate or couverture
- 75 g of cream
- 150 ml of water
- 2 tbsp vanilla sugar
- 2 small espresso
- Cinnamon/sugar

Preparation

Heat the chocolate, cream, water, and sugar in the pot and froth, then place in two tall glasses and gently pour in the espresso. Sprinkle with cinnamon/sugar, and you're done!

Christmas coffee with an orange fragrance

Ingredients

- 600 ml of coffee
- 4 tablespoons cream, beaten
- 2 El Christmas - orange syrup

Preparation

Brew coffee, beat and add cream, and finally flavor with the syrup.

Hot Schokolade in white

Ingredients

- 50 g white chocolate
- 100 ml of cream
- 200 ml of water
- 20 g vanilla sugar

Preparation

Heat 50 ml of cream, water, and chocolate in a saucepan, season to taste with vanilla sugar. Beat 50 ml of cream. Spread the liquid and the cream over two glasses and possibly add a few chocolate sprinkles to the cream

---

Lemon and ginger tea

Ingredients

- gingerroot
- 1 slice of lemon, unsprayed
- 1 tl of candy
- water

Preparation

Slice the ginger, cut off the lemon slice, put both in a glass, and pour over with boiling water. Sweeten and serve with candy.

Mürbchen

Ingredients

- 100g spelled flour Type1050
- 90g margarine, milk-free
- 25g ground almonds
- 1 pack of vanilla sugar
- 30 g of powdered sugar

Preparation

Knead all ingredients to smooth dough. Divide the dough into 16 pieces and shape into balls. Place the balls on a baking tray and press flat with a serving. Bake at 170 degrees for 20 minutes until the cookies on the rim lightly turn brown.

Spiced cookies

Ingredients

- 125 g margarine, milk-free
- 40 g of powdered sugar
- 150 g of flour
- 25 grams of grated coconut
- 1 teaspoon grated orange peel
- 1 Msp. Cinnamon, allspice, cardamom
- 1 pinch of salt

Preparation

Knead all ingredients into dough and shape into a ball. Pack the dough airtight and place in the fridge for 30 minutes to cool. Remove dough from the fridge, pour through and roll out on a floured surface. Cut out biscuits with cookie cutters and place the biscuits on a baking sheet. Bake at 160 degrees convection for about 10 minutes.

Knuspertaler

Ingredients

- 150g margarine, milk-free
- 80g coconut sugar, eg from Agava
- 1 pk vanilla sugar
- 200g of flour
- 1/2 teaspoon salt

Preparation

1. Melt the margarine in a saucepan and let it cool again. Turn creamy with the coconut blossom sugar and the vanilla sugar. Knead the flour and salt together and form the dough into two rolls. If the dough is too crumbly, work with damp fingers and squeeze the rollers firmly. Wrap in cling film and place in the refrigerator for an hour.
2. Slice with a slender knife and place the cookies on a baking sheet covered with baking paper. Bake in a preheated oven at 170 ° C top/bottom heat for about 12 minutes.

Aroma water with rosemary

Ingredients

- 1/2 orange, unsprayed
- 1 sprig of rosemary
- 1 liter of mineral water, cooled

Preparation

Rub the sprig of rosemary between your fingers so that it can deliver its aroma better. Cut the orange into thin slices. Put both in a container and fill with mineral water. Let it rest for 30 minutes.

Chocolate marshmallow cake

Ingredients

- 2 eggs
- 2 egg whites
- 120g sugar
- 150g of flour
- 50g cornstarch
- 10 chocolate kisses
- 500ml cream
- 3 pck

Preparation

1. Separate the eggs and stir the 2 egg yolks with 60g of sugar very frothy. Beat the 4 egg whites until stiff and let the remaining 60g sugar trickle over. Mix flour and cornstarch and sift on the egg yolk cream. Sprinkle with egg whites and fold carefully. Pour the dough into a greased springform pan and bake at 200 ° C (circulating air 160 ° C) for about 20 minutes. Leave to cool on a grid and cut twice across.
2. For the filling, whip cream with a cream stiff. Slightly remove some cream for garnish. Separate the chocolate kisses from the waffles and place under the cream. Fill the cake with the cream and spread it all over. Garnish with cream dab and the waffles.

Vegetable pizza

Ingredients - 6 (1 plate)

- 200g of flour

- 4 tbsp olive oil
- 1/2 pck dry yeast
- 80ml lukewarm water
- 1 tb sugar
- 1/2 tsp salt
- 200g tomatoes, canned
- 1 onion
- 2 tbsp butter
- 200g mushrooms, canned leaves
- 100g corn, canned
- 100g creme fraiche with herbs
- Grated 100g Gouda
- Salt, pepper, oregano

Preparation

1. Mix flour with sugar and yeast. Add water and knead into a smooth dough. Let it go for 45 minutes. Then add the olive oil and salt and knead vigorously. Roll out and place on a baking tray covered with baking paper. Let it go again for 10 minutes.
2. Finely chop the onion and sauté in the butter. Add tomatoes and bring to a boil. If necessary, chop mushrooms and add. Taste and spread on the dough. Spread the crème fraîche with two teaspoons on the pizza. Add corn and grated Gouda.
3. Bake at 200 ° C for about 30 minutes.

Fruity zucchini salad

Ingredients

- 400g zucchini
- 1 small onion
- 4 tbsp olive oil
- 100g pineapple preserve, drained
- Salt, paprika
- thyme

Preparation

Dice the slices and fry in oil until oily. Slice the zucchini and add. Season with salt, paprika, and thyme. Allow to cool and mix with the pineapple cut into pieces.

Chocolate and vanilla cupcakes

Ingredients

- 110g butter
- 150g sugar
- 1 egg
- 200g of flour
- 50g whole milk chocolate
- 1 tbsp soda
- 75g butter
- 175g double cream cheese
- 100g powdered sugar
- 2 pck vanilla sugar

Preparation

1. Melt the milk chocolate. Stir butter and sugar until creamy and stir in the lukewarm, liquid chocolate. Add the egg and then stir in the flour mixed with soda. Spread the mixture on 12 muffin dishes and bake in a preheated oven at 180 ° C (circulating air 160 ° C) for 25 minutes.
2. For the cream, mix soft butter with sifted icing sugar and vanilla sugar until creamy. Stir in the cream cheese and sprinkle the mixture on the cooled muffins.

Lime and coconut cake

Ingredients

- 2 limes
- 300 g of flour
- 2 tbsp soda
- 1 tbsp lime juice
- 160 g of glucose
- salt
- 2 chicken eggs
- 160 g rapeseed oil
- 200 ml of kefir
- 60 grams of grated coconut

Preparation

1. Rub the lime peel, grate the skin thinly on a grater and then squeeze out the lime.
2. Mix flour, baking soda, 100 g glucose and salt in a bowl.
3. Add lime zest, 1 tbsp. Juice, egg, oil and kefir and stir for about 3 minutes.
4. Lay the bottom of a rectangular shape with baking paper. Add dough, smooth and bake in a preheated oven at 200 ° C (gas: stage 3, circulating air 180 ° C) for about 20 minutes.
5. Simmer 60g dextrose, 4l of water and the remaining lime juice for 3 -5 minutes to a syrup.
6. Immediately after baking, pierce the still-hot cake several times with a wooden stick and drizzle the still hot syrup over it. Sprinkle cake with grated coconut, and allow it to cool.

Fish soup

Ingredients

- fish bones and fish
- 150 grams of fish, for example, cod, haddock or fresh salmon
- 1 small leek

- dill and/or parsley

Preparation

1. Put fish bones and fish in a pan with 1 liter of water. Bring this slowly to the boil and let the broth draw for 2.5 hours.
2. Sift the broth.
3. Cut the 150 grams of fish into pieces. Cut the leek into rings and finely chop the herbs.
4. Add the fish, leek, and herbs to the sieved broth. Let it cook for a while.

Sweet rice porridge

Ingredients

- 7½ dl of milk
- 250 g of rice
- 250 g of sugar
- grated zest of 1 lemon
- 1 cinnamon stick
- cinnamon powder
- 3 egg yolks

Preparation

1. Bring the milk to the boil.
2. Add the rice, sugar, lemon zest and cinnamon stick when the milk is boiling.
3. Remove the pan from the heat when the rice is cooked. Remove the cinnamon stick.
4. Allow to cool for 5 minutes.
5. Beat the egg yolks and add them to the rice mixture.
6. Mix everything well together.
7. Place the pan over medium heat and keep it on the boil for 5 to 10 minutes. Be careful that it doesn't matter.
8. Let cool well. Serve cold with some cinnamon powder.

Roast beef roast

Ingredients

- 4 tbsp olive oil
- ¼ tsp dried basil
- ¼ tsp dragon
- pepper
- 250 g roast beef in one piece
- ½ tomato
- ½ root
- ½ medium onion
- ½ celery stick
- 1 clove of garlic
- olive oil for frying
- ¼ glass of red wine

Preparation

1. Mix the 4 tbsp olive oil with the basil, tarragon, and pepper until smooth.
2. Rub the roast beef with this and let it marinate overnight in the fridge.
3. Preheat the oven to 160 - 170 degrees on the day of preparation.
4. Finely chop the tomato, carrot, onion and celery sticks.
5. Heat some olive oil in a frying pan and fry the meat alternately brown in about 3 minutes per side.
6. Grease a baking dish and put the meat in it.
7. Add the tomato mixture and the garlic and pour in the wine and some water.
8. Bake the meat in the oven. In general, the baking time per 500 grams is 30 minutes for medium and 45 minutes for baking. Occasionally pour some of the baking water over the meat.
9. At the end of the cooking time, remove the meat from the baking dish.
10. Puree the vegetables and the cooking liquid and let it reduce by half.

11. Slice the meat and add the sauce.

Gazpacho

Ingredients

- 2 slices of white bread
- 250 g of tomatoes
- ½ bell pepper (green or red)
- ½ cucumber
- ¼ onion
- ½ clove of garlic
- 1 tbsp olive oil
- vinegar to taste

Preparation

1. Cut the crusts off the bread. The crusts are not used. Crumble the rest of the bread.
2. Peel the tomatoes, remove the seeds and cut the rest into small pieces.
3. Mix the tomatoes and the breadcrumbs with a mixer until a smooth cream appears.
4. Cut the bell pepper and cucumber into small pieces and chop the onion finely.
5. Clean the garlic and crush it.
6. Add everything to the tomato mix.
7. Add a little water and mix everything into a smooth thick soup.
8. Add oil and vinegar.
9. Allow the soup to cool well in 2 to 3 hours in the refrigerator.

Couscous salad

Ingredients

- 125 g couscous

- 4 spring onions
- 1 red pepper
- ½ zucchini
- 50 g peas (frozen)
- 1 lemon
- 50 g fresh parsley
- 1 tsp fresh mint
- 1 tbsp fresh coriander
- 5 tbsp olive oil
- pepper

Preparation

1. Prepare the couscous according to the instructions on the package.
2. Allow the couscous to cool.
3. Meanwhile, wash the spring onions and cut into rings.
4. Also, clean the bell pepper and zucchini and cut into small cubes.
5. Cook the peas briefly and drain them.
6. Rinse the green peas with cold water and drain them.
7. Finely chop the fresh herbs.
8. Squeeze the lemon over a large bowl and season with pepper.
9. Add the couscous and all other ingredients and mix everything well.

Pasta with avocado pesto and broccoli

Ingredients

- 200 g (whole grain) pasta
- 300 g broccoli florets
- 1 lemon, waxed
- 1 avocado
- 1 large hand fresh basil (approx. 20 g)
- 2 cloves of garlic
- 25 g pine nuts
- 30 g grated Parmesan cheese

- freshly ground pepper
- 2 tbsp olive oil
- Requirements: food processor or hand blender

Preparation

1. Cook the pasta according to the instructions on the package. When draining the pasta, save ¼ cup of water for the pesto.
2. Cook the broccoli florets in about 8 minutes until done.
3. Grate half a zest of the lemon and squeeze the fruit. Cut the avocado in half, remove the kernel and cut into strips. Spoon the strips out of the peel.
4. In a food processor, add the basil, garlic, pine nuts, Parmesan cheese, zest of half lemon, juice of a whole lemon and some freshly ground pepper. Mix everything well and gradually add the olive oil while mixing and mix until smooth. Then add the avocado and the remaining pasta water. Mix everything well again.
5. Add the sauce to the cooked pasta and stir well so that it is completely covered with the sauce. Finally, add the broccoli to the pasta and serve.

Fish package with cod

Ingredients

- 400 g of rice
- 4 sheets of aluminum foil
- dash of oil
- dash of coconut milk
- 400 g zucchini
- 400 g fennel
- 4 pieces of cod of approximately 100 grams
- 2 tbsp dill
- 2 lemons
- black pepper or 4-season pepper

Preparation

1. Heat the oven to 180 ° C.
2. Cook the rice according to the instructions on the package.
3. Cut the zucchini into cubes and the fennel into slices.
4. Put the aluminum foil down and spread the rice over it with some oil and coconut milk. Place the zucchini and fennel on top and then place the cod on the rice and vegetables. Divide the dill over the packages.
5. Squeeze one of the lemons and cut the other into segments. Divide the juice and the segments over the packages. Add pepper to taste.
6. Fold the packages tightly. (No steam may escape.)
7. Place the packets in the oven for 20-25 minutes (depending on the thickness of the fish).

Spaghetti with kale and meatballs

Ingredients

- 350 g half-to-half minced meat
- 300 g sliced kale
- 1 rusk
- 1 tbsp dried oregano
- 2 tsp Jonnie Boer Picadillo (spice mix)
- 250 g mushrooms in pieces
- 2 tbsp liquid fry & roast
- freshly ground pepper
- 1 onion, chopped
- 300 g (whole grain) spaghetti
- 2 cloves of garlic, chopped
- piece of Parmesan cheese
- 4 sun-dried tomatoes (in oil) in pieces

Preparation

1. Put the minced meat in a bowl, crumble the rusk above it and sprinkle with the spice mix. Knead well together and make small meatballs.
2. Heat the frying pan in a frying pan with a small dash of oil (from the sun-dried tomatoes). Bake the meatballs brown, add a splash of water and cook for about 10 minutes with the lid on the pan. Keep warm with a lid on the pan.
3. Bring a pan of water to the boil for the spaghetti (add the spaghetti later).
4. Heat 2 tablespoons of oil in a wok and fry the onion until it is glassy, then add the garlic and the tomato pieces and fry for 1 minute. Add the kale and stir until it has shrunk. Add a tablespoon of boiling water. Put a lid on the pan and let it simmer for 20 minutes. Add the oregano after 15 minutes.
5. In another frying pan, heat a tablespoon of oil and add the mushrooms with freshly ground pepper. Allow the moisture to evaporate and then bake until golden brown, stirring.
6. Cook the spaghetti at the same time.
7. Spoon the spaghetti and mushrooms into the wok and mix in the kale.
8. Serve the spaghetti with the minced meatballs. Grate some Parmesan cheese on the plate.

Couscous with pumpkin and chickpeas

Ingredients

- 1 bottle squash
- 1 tbsp liquid frying fat
- 2 tbsp honey
- 200 g couscous
- 1 orange, waxed
- 400 g canned chickpeas
- 4 tbsp olive oil
- 2 tsp ras el hanout (for example from Jonnie de Boer or Pure Spices from firm Verstegen)
- 75 g raisins

Preparation

1. Preheat the oven to 200 ° C.
2. Wash the pumpkin and halve the length. Remove the seeds and stringy inside with a spoon. Leave the skin on. Cut both halves into 1 cm cubes.
3. Grease the baking sheet with liquid baking & roasting (or use baking paper).
4. Mix the pumpkin with the honey and spread on the greased baking sheet.
5. Bake the pumpkin in the oven for about 20 minutes until the pumpkin is cooked. Scoop halfway through once.
6. Meanwhile, prepare the couscous according to the instructions on the package.
7. Grate the orange zest of the orange and squeeze the fruit.
8. Drain the chickpeas in a colander and rinse with cold running water.
9. Mix the couscous with orange zest and juice, chickpeas, olive oil, ras el hanout, and raisins.
10. Divide the pumpkin on the couscous

Vegetable spread of broad beans, spinach and bell pepper

Ingredients

- ½ green pepper (about 80 g)
- 1 stem spring onion (about 15 g)
- 130 grams (drained weight) of broad beans
- 100 grams of fresh spinach
- 1 tsp lemon juice
- ½ tsp curry powder
- ½ tsp pepper

Preparation

1. Cut the bell pepper and spring onion into small pieces.
2. Rinse the broad beans under the tap.

3. Combine broad beans, bell pepper and fresh spinach in a large bowl.
4. Puree the ingredients with the hand blender until a smooth mass is created.
5. Add the sliced spring onion.
6. Season the vegetable spread with lemon juice, curry powder, and pepper.
7. Spread a thick layer of vegetable spread on a sandwich or cracker, for example

---

Vegetable spread of carrot, parsnip, and apple

Ingredients

- 200 g of carrots
- 100 g of parsnip
- 1 apple (approximately 135 g) with peel (eg Pink Lady or Elstar)
- ½ tsp pepper
- ½ tsp ground cumin seeds

Preparation

1. Bring a pan of water to the boil.
2. Peel the carrots and parsnip and cut into 1.5 cm pieces.
3. Cook the carrots and parsnip 10 minutes until they are soft.
4. Drain the cooked carrots and parsnip.
5. Cut the apple into small pieces and add it to the carrots and parsnip.
6. Puree with the hand blender until smooth.
7. Add the pepper and cumin seeds to the mixture.
8. Allow the vegetable spread to cool in the refrigerator.
9. Spread a thick layer of vegetable spread on a sandwich or cracker, for example.

Fruit spread with pear and ginger

Ingredients

- 360 g of peeled pears (about 2 pears)
- 3 g fresh ginger root
- 1 tsp lemon juice

Preparation

1. Bring a pan of water to the boil.
2. Meanwhile, peel the pears and cut into 2 cm cubes.
3. Peel and grate the ginger.
4. Boil the pear and ginger for 7 minutes until the pear is soft.
5. Drain the cooked pear and ginger.
6. Put the pear and ginger in a bowl and puree them into compote with a hand blender.
7. Add the lemon juice and stir it into the mixture.
8. Allow the fruit spread to cool in the refrigerator.
9. For example, spread a slice of the fruit spread on a sandwich or cracker.

Overnight Oats

Ingredients

- 40 g (6 tbsp) oatmeal
- 80 ml semi-skimmed milk
- 3 tbsp skyr *
- cinnamon, sugar or honey to taste
- 80 g blueberries from the freezer
- Skyr is yogurt from Iceland. It is for sale under the brand name Arla Skyr, among other things.

Preparation

1. Mix the oatmeal with the milk and then stir in the skyr.
2. Add cinnamon, sugar or honey to taste and then the berries.

3. Put the Overnight Oats in the fridge. Leave it there overnight. (After about 4 hours it tastes great too!)

Spicy pepper mix

Ingredients

- 3 tbsp ground pepper
- 1 tsp ground thyme
- 1 tsp paprika powder
- ½ tsp garlic powder
- ½ tsp onion powder

Preparation

1. Mix all herbs well together.
2. Store the mix in a closed jar in a dark place.

Mexican spice mix

Ingredients

- 2 tsp cayenne pepper
- 3 tsp garlic powder
- 2 tsp cumin
- 1 tsp paprika powder
- 2 tsp oregano

Preparation

1. Mix all herbs well together.
2. Store the mix in a closed jar in a dark place.

Italian spice mix

Ingredients

- 2 tsp basil
- ½ tsp garlic powder
- 1 tsp oregano
- 1 tsp parsley
- ½ tsp thyme

Preparation

1. Mix all herbs well together.
2. Store the mix in a closed jar in a dark place

Indonesian spice mix

Ingredients

- 1 tsp chili
- 1 tsp lemongrass
- 1 tsp ginger
- ½ tsp cinnamon
- 2 tsp garlic powder
- 1 tsp cumin
- 1 tsp coriander
- 1 tsp turmeric

Preparation

1. Mix all herbs well together.
2. Store the mix in a closed jar in a dark place.

Salmon-pasta casserole

Ingredients

- 300 g (fresh) salmon
- 300 g penne rigate
- 300 g of broccoli
- 3 spring onions
- 4 tomatoes
- 200 g of cottage cheese
- 2 - 3 tbsp basil
- 75 g of grated 30+ cheeseless salt
- pinch of lemon pepper (Jonnie Boer)
- low-sodium fish herbs

Preparation

1. Preheat the oven to 200 degrees.
2. Cook the penne in plenty of boiling water according to the package. Cook the broccoli in plenty of water for 10 - 12 minutes until al dente.
3. Meanwhile, cut the spring onions into thin rings and the tomatoes into pieces.
4. Cut the salmon into small cubes, remove sheets and bones and divide the salmon into pieces. Season the salmon with low-sodium fish herbs.
5. Drain the penne and broccoli and mix it with the salmon, spring onion, tomato, cottage cheese, and basil. Season with lemon pepper.
6. Divide the mixture in a low baking dish and sprinkle the grated cheese over it.
7. Let the dish cook in the middle of the preheated oven in about 15 minutes.

Speculaas Tiramisu

Ingredients

- 500 ml whipped cream
- 100 g fine granulated sugar
- 500 g mascarpone
- 2 bags of vanilla sugar
- 1 pack of gingerbread
- mug of espresso, cooled
- cocoa powder for the finish

Preparation

1. Beat the whipped cream with half the sugar and put it in the fridge as long as possible.
2. Mix the mascarpone with the other half of the sugar and the vanilla sugar.
3. Mix whipped cream and mascarpone together, don't beat for too long.
4. Dip the gingerbread cookies 1 by 1 briefly in the coffee and roughly crumble them with a fork in a dish.
5. Put a layer of gingerbread on the bottom of a dish or glasses and then a layer of the mascarpone mixture.
6. Repeat this a number of times.
7. Cover and put it in the refrigerator. Make 1 day or even 2 days in advance.
8. Before serving, cover with a thick layer of cocoa powder (through a sieve).

Cream Gingerbread

Ingredients

- 125g honey
- 125g sugar
- 50 ml of cream
- 225g of flour

- 10g cocoa powder
- 50g spoon biscuit
- 1 tbsp soda
- 1 Tl lemon peel
- 1 Tl gingerbread spice

Preparation

Boil the honey with sugar and cream and cool. Finely grate the spoon biscuit and knead with the remaining ingredients to smooth dough. Cut out any shapes and bake at 180 ° C for about 15 minutes.

Snowflake

Ingredients

- 125g margarine
- 50g powdered sugar
- 1 pck of vanilla sugar
- 50g of flour
- 125g cornstarch
- 20g ground almonds

Preparation

Knead all ingredients and refrigerate for 30 minutes. Form balls out of the dough and press flat with a fork. Place on a baking sheet covered with baking paper and bake at 175 ° C for about 15 minutes. After cooling, dust with icing sugar.

Pear crumble with vanilla sauce

Ingredients

- 4 pears (a 150g)
- 1 tbsp lemon juice

- 100g of flour
- 50g sugar
- 80g butter
- 1 teaspoon cinnamon
- For the vanilla sauce:
- 150ml of water
- 50ml cream
- 1 pck of vanilla sugar
- Go 1 tsp custard powder

Preparation

1. For the crumble, knead the cold butter with flour, sugar, and cinnamon and crumble. Refrigerate for 30 minutes.
2. Cut the pears into small pieces and sprinkle with the lemon juice. Put into a greased casserole dish (or 4 small molds) and sprinkle with the crumbles. Bake in a preheated oven at 180 ° C for about 25 minutes. (For small forms about 20 minutes)
3. For the vanilla sauce, mix all ingredients well with a whisk and bring to a boil while stirring.

Potato Gratin

Ingredients

- 300g boiled potatoes, watered
- 50g leek
- 30g smoked bacon
- 1 cup of crème fraîche with herbs
- 30g Gouda, 48% fat (1 slice)
- 1 tbsp breadcrumbs
- 1 tbsp cold butter

Preparation

Slice the boiled potatoes. Finely chop the bacon and leave in a pan. Add the finely chopped leek rings and steam until soft. Add creme fraiche and stir well. Mix in the potatoes and place in a casserole dish. Cut the Gouda into small cubes and mix with the breadcrumbs. Sprinkle over the gratin and top with butter flakes. Bake at 200 ° C for about 20 minutes.

Rice casserole with cherries

Ingredients

- 300ml of water
- 150 ml of cream
- 1 pck of vanilla sugar
- 100g rice pudding
- 1 egg
- 1 egg white
- 50g butter
- 50g sugar
- 200g sour cherries, canned food dripped off
- 1 tbsp breadcrumbs
- 1 tablespoon of sugar

Preparation

1. Mix water and cream in a saucepan and bring to a boil. Sprinkle the rice pudding and vanilla sugar and cook with occasional stirring on low heat for 25 minutes. Cool lukewarm.
2. Stir the butter with the sugar until creamy and stir in the egg yolk. Beat the egg whites to a stiff snow. Stir rice pudding underneath the fat and fold in the egg whites.
3. Put the cherries in a baking dish and pour in the rice mixture. Sprinkle with sugar and breadcrumbs. Bake at 180 ° C for about 30 minutes.

Poor knight with apple compote

Ingredients

- 4 large (or 8 small) slices of white bread
- 80 ml of cream
- 120ml of water
- 1 egg
- 1 Tl custard powder (for cooking)
- 2 tbsp sugar
- bread crumbs
- 40g butter
- Sugar and cinnamon to taste
- 400g apple compote

Preparation

Mix cream and water and stir with the custard powder, sugar and egg until smooth. Halve or quarter the slices of white bread and turn them in the egg mass. Then turn into breadcrumbs and bake in hot butter until golden brown on both sides. Sprinkle with cinnamon sugar to taste and serve with the apple compote.

Herbal Cupcakes

Ingredients

- 200g of flour
- 2 tbsp soda
- 1 egg
- 150g thin quark
- 2 tbsp olive oil
- 2 tablespoons of chopped parsley
- pinch of salt
- 1 onion
- For the topping
- 200g thin quark

- 1 tablespoon of chives
- 1 tablespoon of chopped parsley
- 100g cream cheese, double cream stage
- Salt pepper

Preparation

1. Finely chop the onion and fry in the olive oil. Let cool. Mix with all other ingredients for the dough with the blender and spread on 12 muffin cups. Bake at 180 ° C (circulating air 160 ° C) for about 20 minutes.
2. Mix cottage cheese with cream cheese, herbs and spices and spread on the muffins.

Filled cannelloni

Ingredients

- 100g canneloni (gross weight)
- 2 tablespoons rapeseed oil
- 100g mushrooms, canned
- 100g zucchini
- 50g spring onion
- 1 egg
- 50g creme fraiche
- Salt, pepper, oregano
- 1 tbsp breadcrumbs
- 1 tbsp butter
- 1 slice of butter cheese (30g)

Preparation

1. Cook the cannelloni in plenty of salted water according to the instructions on the package.
2. For the filling, cut the zucchini and the spring onion into small pieces and fry in the rapeseed oil. Add mushrooms and crème fraiche and season to taste. Allow the mass to cool slightly and

add the egg. Pour into the cannelloni and place in a greased casserole dish. Divide the cheese into small cubes and spread over the cannelloni with the breadcrumbs. Bake for 15 minutes at 200 ° C.

Spicy pancakes with leeks

Ingredients

- 100g of flour
- 1 egg
- 200ml mineral water
- 50ml cream
- 1/2 tbsp soda
- pinch of salt
- 3 rape oil
- 150g leek
- 2 slices of cooked ham (60g)
- 125g creme fraiche with herbs
- black pepper

Preparation

1. From flour, egg, mineral water, cream and soda and salt stir a pancake batter and let rest for 10 minutes. Bake 2 pancakes from the dough in a spoonful of rape oil.
2. Cut the leek into fine rings and steam the canola oil in a spoonful. Cut the ham into strips and stir with the crème fraîche under the leek. Season with black pepper and fill in the pancakes.

Stew with chicken and pumpkin

Ingredients

- 400 g chicken fillet
- 600 g pumpkin

- 200 g green beans
- 3 cloves of garlic
- 1 red chili pepper
- 1 piece of ginger root (50 g)
- 1 can of tomato puree (70 g)
- 1 tbsp coriander (ground)
- 1 tsp cumin (ground)
- 4 tbsp sunflower oil
- 1 can of coconut milk (500 ml)
- 1 hand fresh mint
- 1 hand fresh coriander

Preparation

1. Cut the chicken fillet into strips or cubes of approximately 3 cm. Cut the pumpkin into cubes (or buy them into cubes).
2. Remove the green beans and cook until al dente in 10 minutes.
3. Peel the garlic and halve the cloves.
4. Halve the pepper and remove the seeds (or not if you like spicy).
5. Put the garlic, chili pepper, ginger, tomato puree, ground coriander, and ground cumin in a blender and mix into a spice paste. (You can also use a mortar to make the spice paste; first cut the ingredients into small pieces. More work, but also more taste.)
6. Heat the olive oil in a frying pan, add the spice paste and let it simmer for 5 minutes (do not let it cook).
7. Add the chicken cubes and let the chicken brown on all sides.
8. Pour the coconut milk with the chicken, add the pumpkin cubes and simmer over medium heat with the lid on the pan for 10 to 15 minutes.
9. Warm the green beans for the last few minutes.
10. Chop the fresh mint and coriander. Sprinkle the dish with it.

Waldorf pasta salad

Ingredients

- 300 g chicken fillet

- freshly ground pepper
- paprika powder
- 1 - 2 tbsp olive oil or liquid fry & roast
- 250 g uncooked pasta
- 1/2 head of iceberg lettuce
- 2 small apples
- 3 celery stalks
- 1 bowl of celery salad of 200 grams
- 50 ml low-fat yogurt
- 50 g walnuts

Preparation

1. Sprinkle the chicken fillet with freshly ground pepper and paprika powder.
2. Heat the olive oil or fry in a frying pan. Bake the chicken fillet in 10 - 15 minutes and let the chicken fillet cool.
3. Cut the chicken fillet into slices or cubes.
4. Cook the pasta according to the instructions on the package and let the pasta cool.
5. Cut the iceberg lettuce into thin strips.
6. Peel the apples and cut into 1 cm strips/cubes.
7. Cut the celery into small strips.
8. Carefully mix the pasta, chicken, lettuce, apple, celery, celery salad, and yogurt.
9. Finely chop the walnuts and sprinkle over the meal salad.
10. Season with freshly ground pepper to taste.

Cod from the oven

Ingredients

- 3 tbsp sunflower oil
- 10 g of butter
- 2 onions, cut into rings
- 1 clove of garlic, chopped
- 1 tsp curry powder

- ½ teaspoon ground yellow root (koenjit)
- 4 cod fillets or saithe fillets of 100 grams (thawed)
- freshly ground pepper
- 125 ml sour cream
- 100 g peeled, cooked Dutch shrimps
- 2 tbsp finely chopped dill, tarragon and / or chives

Preparation

1. Spread a thin layer of oil on the inside of a baking dish. Preheat the oven to 200 ° C.
2. Heat the oil and butter in a frying pan and fry the onion rings for a few minutes.
3. Add garlic, curry powder, and koenjit and fry for 1 minute.
4. Spoon the onion mixture into the baking dish.
5. Season the fish with pepper and place the fillets on the onions. Add the sour cream on top.
6. Cover the dish with aluminum foil. Let the fish cook in the oven in about 20 minutes.
7. Divide the shrimp over the fish fillets. Finally, sprinkle the herbs over the dish.

Pak Choy

Ingredients

- 2 shrubs of bok choy with 500 grams
- 2 tbsp sunflower oil
- ¼ red pepper in pieces
- 1 clove of garlic, chopped
- 1 shallot, finely chopped
- 1 scoop of ginger, in pieces
- ginger syrup

Preparation

1. Wash the bok choy and cut the bok choy into 2 cm strips. Keep the stems separate from the leaf.
2. Heat oil in the wok and stir fry the bell pepper, garlic, onion and the sliced paksoist stems for a few minutes.
3. Add the ginger and the pakso leaf and stir-fry for another 2 minutes. Finally, stir the ginger syrup into the vegetables.

Pasta with spinach

Ingredients

- 150 g of spiral macaroni
- 1 onion, chopped
- 2 tablespoons of liquid cooking fat
- 150 g ground beef
- 300 g frozen spinach (eg sub cubes)
- 1 pack of Boursin (80 g)
- freshly ground pepper

Preparation

1. Cook the spiral macaroni according to the instructions on the package.
2. Fry the chopped onion for a few minutes in the liquid baking and roasting fat.
3. Add the minced beef and fry it loose and brown in about 5 minutes.
4. Add the frozen spinach, let it thaw and cook for a few minutes.
5. Add the Boursin and let it melt. Stir well and season with freshly ground pepper.
6. Stir the drained pasta through the spinach mixture and serve immediately.

Broccoli spaghetti with meatballs

Ingredients

- 500 g of broccoli
- 1 onion
- 2 cloves of garlic
- 1 red pepper
- 300 g of spaghetti
- 300 g ground beef
- 100 g grated mature or aged cheese
- 1 egg
- 1 rusk
- 3 tbsp (olive) oil
- 2 tbsp liquid fry & roast
- (freshly ground) black pepper

Preparation

1. Divide the broccoli into small florets and cook until al dente in 7 - 10 minutes. Drain the cooked broccoli in a colander.
2. Cut the onion into small pieces and finely chop the garlic.
3. Cut the red pepper in half, remove the seeds and finely chop the pepper.
4. Cook the spaghetti according to the instructions on the package.
5. Mix the minced meat, grated cheese, half of the red pepper, the egg and the crumbled rusk. Turn the meatballs into small meatballs.
6. Heat 2 tablespoons of liquid fry & roast in a frying pan and fry the meatballs for 10 minutes until brown and cooked.
7. Heat 2 tablespoons (olive) oil in a wok or frying pan and fry the onion and garlic. Then add the broccoli and (stir) fry the whole for a few minutes.
8. Puree or mash the broccoli mixture and mix it with the spaghetti, 1 tablespoon (olive) oil and the rest of the red pepper. Add black pepper to taste (freshly ground).
9. Divide the broccoli spaghetti over 4 plates and place the meatballs on top.

Chicken in coconut sauce

Ingredients

- 2 shallots
- 2 tbsp olive oil
- ½ red chili, chopped
- 1 tbsp honey
- 250 g chicken fillet, in strips
- freshly ground pepper
- grated zest of ½ lemon
- 1 tbsp lemon juice
- 200 ml coconut milk
- cornflour
- chopped parsley

Preparation

1. Chop the shallots and fry them, together with the finely chopped pepper, in the olive oil until light brown.
2. Add the honey and let it caramelize slightly.
3. Add the strips of chicken fillet and fry this.
4. Add freshly ground pepper.
5. Add the lemon zest and lemon juice.
6. Pour the coconut milk into the pan and let the chicken simmer for 10 minutes.
7. Tie the sauce with diluted cornflour.
8. Stir in the finely chopped parsley.

Tagliatelle with Boursin

Ingredients

- 150 g ribbon macaroni
- 2 onions
- 2 tbsp butter

- 200 g mushrooms
- 80 g Boursin
- 2 tbsp whipped cream
- parsley

Preparation

Cook the tagliatelle until done.

1. Fry the chopped onion in the hot butter.
2. Add the sliced mushrooms and fry for about 3 minutes. Remove the pan from the heat.
3. Add the Boursin and the cream and stir until the Boursin has melted.
4. Add the ribbon macaroni and heat through.
5. Sprinkle the finely chopped parsley.

Leek pie

Ingredients

- 6 slices of frozen puff pastry, thawed
- 450 g cleaned leek
- 2 eggs
- 2 tbsp flour
- 125 ml of crème fraiche
- pepper, nutmeg

Preparation

1. Place the thawed slices of dough on top of each other and roll them out into a round piece.
2. Cover the greased baking pan with this and pierce a few holes in the dough.
3. Bake the dough base for about 10 minutes in the middle of a preheated oven at 225 degrees Celsius. Leave the oven on.

4. Cook the leek cut into rings for about 10 minutes and then drain the vegetables well. Beat the eggs with the flour, crème fraîche, pepper and nutmeg.
5. Spoon the leek into the dough bottom and pour the egg mixture over it.
6. Bake the cake in the center of the oven for about 25 minutes until lightly browned and cooked.

Capuchin from Bali

Ingredients

- 100 g capuchins (= 300 g cooked)
- 4 tbsp oil
- 2 cloves of garlic
- 2 onions
- 100 g of cleaned white cabbage
- piece of leek
- 1 tsp sambal
- 100 g bean sprouts
- 2 balls of stem ginger
- celery

Preparation

1. Place the Capuchin the evening before with plenty of water during the week.
2. Drain the weekly water.
3. Put the capuchins on with fresh water and let them simmer for about 1 hour.
4. In the meantime, fry the pressed garlic and the finely chopped onion in the oil. After a few minutes, add the sliced cabbage, as well as the sliced leek and the sambal.
5. Bake for about 10 minutes while stirring. Then add the bean sprouts and the finely chopped ginger and let them warm.
6. Add the capuchins and finally sprinkle finely chopped celery.

Chicken curry with brown rice

Ingredients

- 400 g of brown rice
- 400 g chicken fillet
- 250 g chestnut mushrooms
- 300 g snow peas
- 1 onion
- 350 g pieces of pineapple
- 150 ml of crème fraiche
- 2 tsp curry powder
- pepper to taste

Preparation

1. Cook the rice according to the package.
2. Cut the chicken fillet into cubes and season with some pepper.
3. Clean and halve the mushrooms. Chop the onion.
4. Depilate the snow peas and cook until al dente in 5 minutes.
5. Heat the oil in a frying pan and fry the onion.
6. Turn up the heat, add the chicken and mushrooms and stir-fry.
7. When the chicken is cooked, add the crème fraîche and then stir in the curry powder.
8. Finally, add the pineapple and snow peas and heat this for a while.

Ricotta spread

Ingredients

- 250 g ricotta
- 2 cloves of garlic
- grated zest of a ½ lemon
- 1 tbsp lemon juice
- freshly ground pepper

Preparation

1. Squeeze 2 cloves of (fresh) garlic over the ricotta.
2. Add the grated zest (yellow only) of ½ lemon and 1 tablespoon lemon juice.
3. Add (quite a bit) freshly ground pepper to taste.

ANTI-INFLAMMATORY DIET FOR BEGINNERS

The Complete Guide to Eliminate Inflammation, Revitalizing your Health and Losing Weight with Easy Recipes

Lewis W. Martin

CHAPTER 1: The Origins of The Anti-Inflammatory Diet

Several authors have proposed diets with anti-inflammatory potential, including Dr. Andrew Weil, who is certainly one of the biggest promoters of this diet, like Dr. David Servan-Schreiber and, more recently, Dr. Serfaty-Lacrosniere. They, like many other researchers and health professionals, believe that too much inflammation is one of the common causes of many diseases, including cardiovascular disease, diabetes, and some cancers.

The main principles of the anti-inflammatory diet
The anti-inflammatory diet aims to reduce inflammation in the body which results in different symptoms. It can be considered that this scheme aims to:
- Protect the immune system.
- Help the organization resist and adapt to change.
- Reduce the risk of diseases with an inflammatory component (cardiovascular diseases, asthma, Alzheimer's disease, irritable bowel syndrome, cancer, autoimmune diseases, etc.).
- Increase life expectancy in health.

Authorized foods
This diet is very close to the Mediterranean diet, it consumes a maximum of foods from the plant kingdom, oily fish and not to eat processed foods.
Some authors also advocate reducing the consumption of allergenic foods such as eggs, wheat, peanuts, corn, soy, and dairy products.

How Anti-inflammatory Diet Helps Reduce Chronic Inflammation
The antioxidants contained in fruits and vegetables will help slow down cellular aging and promote a good general condition. At the same time, the omega 3s brought by oleaginous fruits and oily fish will prevent cardiovascular diseases, especially with the decrease in

the consumption of red meat.

Homemade dishes will have the advantage of containing less salt, fats and hidden sugars than commercially processed products and will also contribute to the reduction of inflammatory markers.

One-day type menu with an anti-inflammatory diet
Breakfast
- Cereal Bread
- Tofu Scrambled with
- Orange Turmeric

Lunch
- Lentil salad with tomatoes and mushrooms
- Dark chocolate square
- Green tea

Collation
- Roasted soybeans

Having dinner
- Salmon
- Steak Rice
- Asparagus
- 1 glass of red wine

The advantages and disadvantages of the anti-inflammatory diet
Advantages
- **Satiating**

No problem of satiety with this diet composed of complete foods, the present fibers and the proteins of good nutritional quality allow being well satisfied.
- **Prevention of cardiovascular disease**

With the consumption of good fats, specifically omega 3 and the reduction of saturated fatty acids in red meat, this diet helps prevent cardiovascular disease easily.
- **Respected food balance**

This diet is in line with most international nutrition recommendations, increasing fiber intake through the consumption of fruits and vegetables and whole grains while reducing its intake of red meat and processed products.

Disadvantage
- **May disrupt intestinal transit**

For those unaccustomed to consuming fiber, this diet can disrupt digestion by leading to minor transit and digestive disorders.

CHAPTER 2: What Is Inflammation and What Causes It?

Through inflammation, the body tries to protect itself from tissue and cell damage from all sorts of pathogenic factors. When something harmful and annoying interferes with our body, the natural biological response is its attempt to eliminate it in order to start healing processes.

Inflammation does not exactly mean infection, even when the inflammation itself has led to an infection. The infection can be caused by a virus, bacterium or fungus, and inflammation is the body's response to that infection.

Inflammation is the body's immune response, which is good. However, inflammation can sometimes lead to additional inflammation, which can lead to various complications.

The classic symptoms of inflammation are:
- Warmth
- Redness
- Swelling
- Pain
- Function malfunction

Inflammation helps wounds heal

By swelling, for example, the body tries to heal itself. Without inflammation, infections and wounds could not be treated. However, it is certainly necessary for this symptom to be properly treated by the doctor in order to avoid further complications.

The inflammation occurs in several stages. The first phase is damaging, and the negative consequences of this development very quickly. For this reason, the damaging phase is difficult to distinguish from the second phase - the so-called escalation phase, which is the result of a disturbance in the microcirculation. In other words, the first stage of inflammation occurs with irritation, which immediately goes on to inflammation. Inflammation is followed by suppuration.

Neurologists at the Ohio Clinic have found that inflammation actually heals and aids damaged muscle tissue. According to scientists, this finding may lead to new and different from existing therapies for acute muscular trauma. They are adamant that inflammation, as part of our innate immunity naturally inherent in the human body, is an absolutely necessary 'evil.' This immunity has nothing to do with the so-called adaptive immunity acquired over time, after vaccination or other external factors. This means that inflammation is part of the mechanisms of innate immunity.

What is the difference between chronic inflammation and acute inflammation?
Acute inflammation develops and complicates rapidly. The signs and symptoms of acute inflammation are present over a period of days, and very rarely, the process can take weeks or months.
Diseases and conditions that can lead to acute inflammation can be acute bronchitis, nail ingrowth, a sore throat caused by cold or flu, skin wounds, acute appendicitis, dermatitis, acute tonsillitis, acute infectious meningitis, acute sinusitis, blow.
Chronic inflammation is a process that has gone on for a very long time, which means months or even years. In most cases, it results from poorly treated acute inflammation, but can also develop when the immune system attacks healthy tissues and more.

What is happening in our body - inflammation or infection?

Throughout life, the human body undergoes a number of inflammations. We are used to considering them as infectious. Medical professionals are adamant that there is a significant difference, and it is good to know each other to be alert when we have a problem.
Our wound can become inflamed, and it is a completely natural process of our body, whereas if it is infected, the culprits here will be certain viruses, fungi, or bacteria. In inflammation, we do not always necessarily talk about infection. That is why it is appropriate to be aware and not to sign equality between the two.

When the inflammation occurs

Our body has several lines of defence that it activates under the necessary risk conditions. When we have an irritant in the form of pathogens 1 or disease-carrying microorganisms, it is perfectly normal for white blood cells to activate our innate immunity and respond with inflammation.

This means that everything is fine with us, and we are fighting the external cause. If our immune system had collapsed, the consequences would be more serious, even fatal. In the place of the affected cells or tissues, inflammation sets in, precisely to repair them, but also to prevent the spread of the damage to healthy organs nearby.

Any environmental factor that has the ability to jump over our adaptation and defence potential can provoke inflammation. And it is divided into several phases, the signs being quickly and easily recognizable. First, the pain is catching up, followed by local warming, oedema, and the skin becomes red, and functional disorders occur.

In the area, the blood increases in quantity, and therefore it results in warming and redness. Swelling is a symptom of retained body fluids. Irritation of the nerve endings is impossible to avoid at this point, and through pain, the body signals us that it is in danger.

Stages of inflammation

Tissue damage is the initial step that causes all other unpleasant consequences. From there on, the mediators, which are special compounds, have their say. They separate in the space between the cells and affect the permeability of their membranes. Among the main mediators is histamine, whose action is observed in the initial manifestations of inflammation. It clears the passage of leukocytes that deal with pathogens.

Another mediator is serotonin, which comes from platelets and affects the amount of blood flow. Cytokines, they also take care of oedema by directing white blood cells to the inflamed area and also signalling the bone marrow to produce more leukocytes. Their action is also associated with causing temperature, but it is also an integral part of the blood coagulation system, without which inflammation would spread over a larger area and damage surrounding tissues.

In the next phase, the gradual recovery has already started, which is not guaranteed to be complete, but at least will provide partial healing. Once it is over, the moment of scar formation comes. They are not always noticeable from afar, and they may not even be visible when viewed in detail. However, the structure has changed, and, under a microscope, it fades immediately. It is no coincidence that in people who have had heart attacks, doctors have no problem indicating how many they were - the heart also forms scars.

The inflammation itself could be acute or chronic. It is important to differentiate them, not only because of the specific speed at which they are going but also in relation to the particular treatment to be administered. In chronic inflammation, we are talking about a permanent change in the cells, which may not manifest with the characteristic acute signs - high fever, swelling, severe pain.

Help with inflammation

If you have inflammation, you will most likely be prescribed non-steroidal agents and corticosteroids for therapy. However, their side effects are by no means desirable. It is possible to cause damage to the stomach, causing an ulcer, to reduce the function of the immune system, to affect the liver and others.

Some herbs have the ability to reduce and limit inflammation. The Devil's Nail, a plant that comes from Africa, is often used in arthritis, fever, and as a substitute for some painkillers. In ancient times, ginger was used in abdominal disorders, pain due to rheumatoid problems, colic.

Recently, scientists believe that it directly attacks the inflammation of the colon. Turmeric, which is also a member of the ginger family, is another recommended herb for inflammation, arthritis, and even Alzheimer's syndrome.

CHAPTER 3: Lists of Anti-Inflammatory Foods

Most Powerful Anti-Inflammatory Foods

Little or gradual modifications are typically sustainable, more suitable for the body to adjust to, and may decrease your chances of responding to your old habits. Then instead of emptying your locker, including setting out for the Mediterranean, you can start a small step at a point and begin an anti-inflammatory diet.

By appending anti-inflammatory diets that fight inflammation to your diet, you can start to repair your body outwardly, making any sharp differences by regaining health at the cellular level. When you discover foods that heal your body also satisfy your taste buds, you can eliminate the wrong foods that create inflammation without feeling guilty. Let's get a look at 15 of the best anti-inflammatory foods you can combine to your diet.

1. Green Leafy Vegetables
It is the principal food you require to fill your refrigerator when combating inflammation. Fruits and the vegetables are wealthy in antioxidants that restore cellular health as well as anti-inflammatory flavonoids. If you have complexity eating green leafy vegetables, you can make anti-inflammatory vegetable juices where you can merge greens.

For instance, when you consume biceps, it is abundant in antioxidant vitamins A plus C and vitamin K, which can defend your brain upon oxidative stress induced by free radical damage. Consuming biceps can also shield you from vitamin K deficiency.

2. Bok Choy (Chinese cabbage)
Bok choy, also known as Chinese cabbage, is an excellent source of antioxidant vitamins and minerals. Recent research shows that bok choy also contains more than 70 antioxidant phenolic substances. These include acids called hydroxycinnamic, which are robust antioxidants that remove free radicals. As a versatile vegetable, bok

choy can be used in many dishes outside of Chinese cuisine, so it is one of the best anti-inflammatory foods.

3. Celery
The benefits of celery in recent pharmacological research include antioxidant and anti-inflammatory properties, as well as preventing heart disease, which helps improve blood pressure and cholesterol levels. Celery seeds (whole seed form, extract form) have impressive health benefits in itself to reduce inflammation and fight bacterial infections. It is an excellent source of antioxidants and vitamins as well as potassium.

Also, balance is the key to a healthy body without inflammation. An excellent example of inflammation-related mineral balance is celery, the right mix of sodium and potassium-rich foods. Sodium brings liquids and nutrients, while potassium removes toxins. We know that sodium in processed foods is high, but our usual diets are not rich in potassium. Without this pairing, toxins can accumulate in the body and cause inflammation once again. One of the benefits of celery is an excellent source of potassium, as well as antioxidants and vitamins.

4. Beetroot
The most evident marker of food full of antioxidants is its deep color. The umbrella category of antioxidants contains a large number of substances. In general, they fight to repair cell damage caused by inflammation. The beet gives the signature color of antioxidant betalain and is an excellent anti-inflammatory. Among the benefits of beet when added to the diet, we can see that it increases the levels of potassium and magnesium that fight cell repair and inflammation.

Beets also contain a small amount of magnesium, and magnesium deficiency is strongly associated with inflammation conditions. While calcium is a vital nutrient, it cannot function well without magnesium in the body. Accumulation of calcium in the body is undesirable. This unpleasant build-up invites, for example, limescale kidney stones, followed by inflammation. However, when a balanced diet is done, calcium-rich anti-inflammatory foods, as well as magnesium, allow the body to better process what is consumed.

5. Broccoli
It is no mystery that broccoli is a worthy addition to either diet, the perfect vegetable for healthful eating. It is valuable for the anti-inflammatory diet. Broccoli is excellent in both potassium and the magnesium, including its antioxidants, which are expressly potent anti-inflammatory factors.

Broccoli holds essential vitamins, flavonoids, and carotenoids and is a significant root of antioxidant power. They go together to decrease oxidative stress inside the body and to inhibit chronic inflammation, including cancer development.

6. Blueberries
In particular, quercetin, which is also found in blueberries, appears as an antioxidant and a powerful anti-inflammatory (the pigments found in some plants). Quercetin, which is found in citrus, olive oil, and dark fruits, is a flavonoid (a useful substance or phytonutrient that is common in fresh foods) that fights inflammation and even cancer. The presence of quercetin is one of the health benefits of blueberries. In a study seeking IBD treatment, noni fruit extract was used to influence intestinal flora and colon damage by inflammatory diseases. Due to the effects of the extract, quercetin produced significant anti-inflammatory effects.

In another study, they found that consuming more blueberries slowed down cognitive decline and improved memory and motor functions. Scientists in this study believed that these results were due to blueberry antioxidants, which prevent the body from oxidative stress and reduce inflammation.

7. Pineapple
Generally, when taken as a supplement, quercetin is coupled with bromelain, a digestive enzyme, which is one of the benefits of pineapple. After years of use as part of an anti-inflammatory food protocol, bromelain is observed to have immune modulation capabilities - i.e., it helps to regulate the immune response that generates unwanted and unnecessary inflammation.

Pineapple also helps to improve heart health because it contains an active bromelain enzyme. Pineapple is the nature's answer to those who struggle with blood clotting and take an aspirin a day for those who want to reduce the risk of a heart attack. Bromelain has been found to stop blood platelets from sticking together or accumulating on the walls of blood vessels (known causes of heart attacks or strokes).

The benefits of pineapple, high in addition to other disease-specific antioxidants that help prevent the formation of vitamin C, vitamin B1, potassium, and manganese supply. Pineapple is full of phytonutrients (plant nutrients), which are useful in addition to many medicines to reduce the symptoms of some of the most common diseases we see today.

8. Salmon Fish
Salmon is an outstanding source of indispensable fatty acids, and it is estimated one of the most fabulous omega-3 foods. The omega-3 is the joint active anti-inflammatory agent that demonstrates consistently decreasing inflammation, including reducing the requirement for anti-inflammatory drugs.

The analysis explains that omega-3 fatty acids decrease inflammation as well as reduce the risk of persistent diseases like heart disease, skin cancer, and arthritis. Omega-3 fatty acids remain concentrated inside the brain and are necessary for cognitive and behavioral function.

Between anti-inflammatory foods, fish and meat are essential components. One of the risks of farm fish is that they do not include the same nutrients as naturally fed fish.

9. Bone Water
Bone juices contain minerals in forms that your body can easily absorb; calcium, magnesium, phosphorus, silicon, sulfur, and others. These include chondroitin sulfates and glucosamine. It is used as additional substances to reduce inflammation, arthritis, and joint pain. When patients suffer from leaking bowel syndrome, they are advised to consume a large number of bone waters containing collagen and amino acid proline and glycine, which may help to improve the damaged cell walls of the leaking intestine and the inflammatory bowel.

10. Walnut
When you follow a diet that does not have a lot of meat, nuts, and

seeds meet your protein and omega-3 needs. To get anti-inflammatory nutrients, you can add omega-3 rich walnuts to green leafy salads with plenty of olive oil, or you can eat a handful of walnuts between meals. Phytonutrients help prevent metabolic syndrome, cardiovascular problems, and type 2 diabetes. Some plant nutrients in walnuts are not found in other foods.

11. Coconut Oil
Much can be written about how herbs and oils work together to form anti-inflammatory partnerships. Lipids (oils) and spices are strong anti-inflammatory compounds, especially coconut oil and turmeric components. A study in India found that antioxidants in coconut oil reduce high levels of inflammation and improve arthritis more quickly than medical drugs.

In addition, oxidative stress and free radicals are the two main causes of osteoporosis. Coconut oil is a leading natural cure for osteoporosis because its benefits include combating such free radicals with high levels of antioxidants.

The use of coconut oil, you can easily use in the kitchen as well as topical preparations. As heat-resistant oil, it is an excellent choice for sauteed anti-inflammatory vegetables.

12. Chia Seed
Fatty acids found in nature are more balanced in our typical diets than those we usually consume. For example, Chia seeds contain omega-3 and omega-6, which should be consumed with each other.

Chia contains essential fatty acids alpha-linolenic and linoleic acid, mucin, strontium, minerals containing vitamins A, B, E and D, antioxidants containing sulfur, iron, iodine, magnesium, manganese, niacin, and thiamine.

Chia is seeds that can reverse inflammation, regulate cholesterol, and lower blood pressure, which is incredibly beneficial for heart health. Also, by reversing oxidative stress, one is less likely to develop atherosclerosis while regularly consuming chia seeds.

13. Flax Seed
Flaxseed, an excellent source of omega-3 and phytonutrients, is full of antioxidants. Lignans are unique fiber-related polyphenols that

provide antioxidant benefits for anti-aging, hormone balance, and cellular health. Polyphenols promote the growth of probiotics in the intestine and may also help eliminate yeast and Candida Fungus in the body.

Before using flaxseed with your anti-inflammatory foods, grind it in a mill to ensure that your digestive system can easily access the benefits of the seeds.

14. Turmeric

The prime component of turmeric is curcumin, an active anti-inflammatory Ingredients. Turmeric, documented its impacts against inflammation in several cases, has confirmed to be invaluable in anti-inflammatory nutrition.

While curcumin is among the significant anti-inflammatory and anti-proliferative agents within the world, aspirin (Bayer, etc.), and ibuprofen (Advil, Motrin, and so on.) have been discovered to have no sound effects.

Because of its noble anti-inflammatory qualities, turmeric is extremely useful in assisting people to treat rheumatoid arthritis (RA). A study from Japan assessed its correlation with interleukin (IL), an inflammatory cytokine identified to be connected in the RA process. It found that lead "significantly decreased these markers of inflammation.

15. Ginger

Used in fresh, dried or extracts, ginger is another immune modulator that helps reduce inflammation caused by overactive immune responses.

Ayurvedic medicine has revealed that ginger can improve the immune system before the recorded date. Ginger is believed to be effective in increasing your body temperature, helping to disperse toxin accumulation in your organs. It is known that our body is good at cleaning the lymphatic system, which is the sewer system.

Ginger's health benefits include reducing inflammation in allergic and asthma diseases.

Inflammatory Foods to Avoid

When you diet with anti-inflammatory foods, you naturally begin to eliminate pro-inflammatory foods and substances. There is nothing as satisfying as a diet rich in whole foods.

The primary suspects are saturated and trans fatty acids. These fats in processed foods increase inflammation and risk factors for obesity, diabetes, and heart disease.

Omega-6 oils that exceed the balance of omega-3 create inflammation in the body. Unfortunately, the University of Maryland Medical Center says, "A typical diet contains 14-25 times more omega-6 fatty acids than omega-3 fatty acids.

Simple, refined sugars and carbohydrates are more culprits than foods that cause inflammation. Limiting refined foods is an essential factor in an anti-inflammatory diet. All grains can replace refined carbohydrates because whole grains are essential food sources. By using fermented yeasts, you can break down nutrients and gain better access to the body.

Also, establishing a regular physical activity routine can help prevent the occurrence or recurrence of systemic inflammation. An active life that is activated by anti-inflammatory foods and is not limited to processed toxic compounds can lead you to free you from inflammation.

CHAPTER 4: What is an anti-inflammatory diet?

An anti-inflammatory diet is a nutrition plan designed to prevent or reduce chronic inflammation. In this case, of course, we are talking about a low degree of severity. Otherwise, you will need a doctor.
Inflammation in our body often occurs as a result of high levels of stress, lack of exercise, chronic inflammation (the immune system releases chemicals designed to fight injuries, bacterial and viral infections, etc.)
It is believed that this diet helps prevent or reduce the manifestations of allergies, Alzheimer's disease, arthritis, asthma, cancer, depression, diabetes, gout, inflammatory bowel disease, irritable bowel syndrome. Also, a similar diet will be useful to those who recover from an injury or surgery.
A typical anti-inflammatory diet consists of fruits, vegetables, low-fat protein, nuts, seeds, and other healthy fats.
Diet, in its essence, is not much different from a healthy diet, to which we are used. Fresher, less fried, whole foods, variety, less sugar.

Tips for following an anti-inflammatory diet:
- Drink plenty of clean water and tea
- Limit your intake of foods high in omega-6 fatty acids (meat, dairy, margarine, corn, sunflower, soy, peanut butter) while increasing your intake of foods rich in omega-3 fatty acids (flaxseed, walnuts, fatty fish)
- Replace red meat with healthier protein sources such as lean poultry, fish, soybeans, beans, and lentils.
- Change margarine and vegetable oils for more healthy fats found in olive oil, nuts, and seeds. Omega-3 fatty acids reduce inflammation, and Omega-6 stimulate. For a healthy person, a balance of both fatty acids is important, but with inflammation, it is recommended to reduce the amount of omega-6
- Instead of peeled grains, choose fibre-rich whole grains such as oats, quinoa, unpolished rice, whole bread, and pasta

- Reduce salt; use anti-inflammatory seasonings such as garlic, ginger, and turmeric for taste
- Eat five to nine servings of antioxidant-rich fruits and vegetables every day.

High antioxidant foods:
- Berries (blueberries, raspberries, blackberries)
- Sweet cherry
- The apples
- Artichokes
- Avocado
- Dark green leafy vegetables (cabbage, spinach, and greens)
- Sweet potato
- Broccoli
- Nuts (such as walnuts, almonds, hazelnuts)
- Beans
- Whole grains (e.g., oats and brown rice)
- Dark chocolate (at least 70 per cent cocoa)

This diet as a whole is suitable for any person since its basis is a healthy diet. In particular, it is recommended to observe it in case of inflammatory processes or suspicion of them. In any case, consult with your doctor first.

CHAPTER 5: Anti-Inflammatory Foods and Their Health Benefits

Proper nutrition is important to maintain the full functioning of the body and can even help prevent disease. In this context, anti-inflammatory foods play a key role and help to reduce health problems and improve the immune system.

With the help of nutritionist of the Equilibrium Therapeutic Center, we have made a list of 10 anti-inflammatory foods and their benefits. The nutritionist warns that to work properly, products must be part of the daily diet, since "sporadic use will not have the desired effect."

Foods with anti-inflammatory action

Thinking about their consumption, the products presented by the nutritionist have in common the ease of being included in daily meals. There are options that can be made in the form of juices, teas, and vitamins. Others may integrate recipes through seasoning or even chocolates. See the list below.

- **Ginger**

Ginger is an ally in fighting diseases such as diabetes and obesity. It can be used in many ways. Ginger is widely used to combat diabetes and obesity.it has a compound known as gingerol, which is responsible for the anti-inflammatory effect. "This substance that gives this spice a spicy flavour. It can be used in the form of teas and juices as a spice" says the nutritionist.

- **Turmeric**

According to the nutritionist, turmeric acts as a barrier, whose goal is to prevent the action of inflammatory agents. The spice acts mainly in the fight against heart disease, diabetes, and even cancer. Turmeric acts as a barrier, blocking inflammation and, like ginger, can be used fresh or powdered.

- **Grape**

A substance called resveratrol, present in the peel and seeds of the fruit has strong anti-inflammatory action. Found mainly in the skin and seeds of red grapes, a substance called resveratrol is responsible for the anti-inflammatory action of the fruit. "In addition to diabetes prevention and weight loss aid, it also has protective action against ultraviolet radiation.

- **Cocoa**

Cocoa has polyphenols in its composition, properties that help fight inflammation. Cocoa helps improve cardiovascular health and has anticarcinogenic action. Polyphenols are the substances in food that fight inflammation.

- **Red Fruits**

Berries, or simply red fruits, are rich in antioxidants and vitamin C, yet work against inflammation. Berries, also known as wild fruits or berries, are rich in antioxidants, vitamin C, procyanidin, and flavonoids, which are important anti-inflammatory properties.

- **Fish**

Cold and deep-water fish, such as salmon, are sources of omega 3, which helps reduce disease risks. Fish such as salmon, tuna, herring, sardines, and horsetail, which are both deep and cold water, are great ways to achieve omega 3, a component famous for aiding weight loss and improving cardiovascular health.

- **Extra Virgin Olive Oil**

Extra virgin olive oils have anti-inflammatory action similar to medicines, ensures nutritionist. The properties of this type of olive oil are so good that they can have the same benefits as a medicine. "Extra virgin olive oil has a substance that inhibits the activity of enzymes involved in inflammation in the same way that some anti-inflammatory drugs work," explains by an expert.

- **Avocado**

Common in vitamins and Mexican dishes, avocado also helps lower cholesterol. Commonly used to make vitamins, the fruit has beta-sitosterol, an anti-inflammatory substance that also contributes to lowering cholesterol levels.

- **Rich flaxseed**

Flaxseed is rich in omega 3 and fibre and helps to have regulated hormones and is a good choice against inflammation. Like fish, rich flaxseed is a source of omega 3 and also helps regulate hormones. "It is high in fibre, contributing to intestinal and heart health and weight control.

- **Garlic**

An important ally of the immune system, garlic has an anti-inflammatory substance in its components. To close our list, allicin, an abiotic compound present in garlic has anti-inflammatory action. In addition, spice enhances the immune system and even protects cardiovascular health. In order for anti-inflammatory foods to be able to protect your body, it is important to invest in food reeducation. "Too much high-glycemic, low-fibre, high-fat Trans foods leads to overproduction of pro-inflammatory mediators, increasing the incidence of chronic disease," "A diet that peels more and unpacks less seems to be the secret to an active immune system.

- **Linseed**

Regular consumption of flaxseed helps protect against bacteria and viruses, thanks to omega 3, plant lignins and phytosterols, and bioflavonoids. Its anti-inflammatory effects are still important to alleviate the symptoms of bronchitis and cystitis and to assist in cases of inflammation of the kidneys and bladder and in respiratory diseases such as asthma.

- **Semisweet chocolate**

Look for brands that contain at least 70% cocoa in the composition. It is the healthiest option because it contains many nutrients such as flavonoids, components that destroy free radicals and help reduce chronic inflammation.

- **Shitake**

The mushroom has polysaccharides that help boost the immune response, which is important for fighting infection. The food also has antimicrobial action.

CHAPTER 6: Simple techniques to fight inflammation

Watch your weight
In addition to rounding the waist and forming the saddlebags, fat cells stimulate the production of harmful proteins that promote inflammation.
- In a study of 16,000 adults, researchers found that obese men were twice as likely as others to have high levels of inflammatory protein, and obese women six times more.
- Many scientists today believe that the increased susceptibility to heart disease and diabetes in overweight people is in part due to inflammation.
- Fortunately, it seems that losing weight can correct the problem.

Replace omega-6 with omega-3
Saturated fats from parsley fat and whole milk contain arachidonic acid, an omega-6 that the body uses to make inflammatory proteins.
- People whose diets are high in saturated fat usually accumulate excess weight in the waist (apple-shaped silhouette).
- However, according to studies in animals and humans, abdominal fat is the one that causes the most inflammation.
- This is another reason for overweight people to consume more fish and flaxseeds: various studies have shown that the consumption of omega-3 lowers levels of inflammatory substances.

Choose your carbohydrates wisely
Recent discoveries by carbohydrate researchers have shed light on their complex and controversial role.
- Many foods contain carbohydrates, and in some cases, these fight inflammation; in others, they aggravate it.
- Once you understand a number of simple concepts, it's easy to choose carbohydrates that hinder inflammation.

Increase your consumption of fruits and vegetables

Could it be that by eating a simple dish of carrots at the meal, we succeed in mitigating chronic inflammation? Yes.

- Fruits and vegetables are the best sources of antioxidants. These substances neutralize the effects of free radicals, natural molecules that attack healthy cells.
- However, the body reacts to the damage of free radicals as it would for any other injury: by inflammation. If we do not eat enough antioxidants, it will get worse.
- For example, British researchers have shown that blood levels of CRP are twice as high among men who consume less vitamin C than those whose diet provides them with an abundance of vitamin C.
- German researchers found that people who went from two to eight servings of fruits and vegetables daily saw their CRP levels fall by one-third in 4 weeks. According to them, this effect was mainly attributable to the carotenoids of vegetables such as carrots, tomatoes, and red peppers.

Brush your teeth after meals
Do not forget to brush your teeth after each meal and floss regularly. In fact, gingivitis disperses inflammation throughout the body, increasing the risk of heart disease and diabetes.

CHAPTER 7: Lists of Anti-Inflammatory Recipes

1. Tuna Tartare with Avocado and Sesame

Preparation time: 1 hour
You will need this for 2 tuna tartare with avocado and sesame

Ingredients
- 300 gr fresh tuna
- 1/2 red onion - chopped
- 1 avocado
- Juice of a lemon slice
- 1 tsp. of sesame oil
- 1 tbsp. roasted sesame seeds + extra for it
- Few sprigs of fresh dill
- 2 tsps. sour cream

Optional: 4 toasted slices of baguette for it

Preparation
1. Cut the tuna into very small cubes. Do the same with the avocado.
2. Take a large bowl and then mix the tuna, avocado, lemon juice, sesame seeds, red onion and sesame oil — season with a pinch of pepper and salt.
3. Place the ring on a plate and add half of the tuna mixture. Press with a spoon and carefully slide the ring off. Make the second steak tart as well.
4. Sprinkle some sesame seeds over the tartare and close with a teaspoon of sour cream and dill on each tuna tartare.

Nutritional Information - Composition Amount (g) CDR (%)
Calories: 219
Total Fat: 12.3g, 19%
Saturated Fat: 6.4g, 32%
Polyunsaturated Fat: 3g

Monounsaturated Fat: 1.8g
Cholesterol: 42.9mg, 14%
Sodium: 227.9mg, 9%
Potassium: 598.3mg
Total Carbohydrate: 5.4g, 2%
Dietary Fiber: 2.6g, 10%
Sugars: 1g
Protein: 22g
Vitamin A: 1.7%
Vitamin C: 6.6%
Calcium: 5%
Iron: 7.7%

2. Herb omelet with smoked salmon

Preparation Time: 15 minutes

Ingredients for 4 portions
- One cucumber
- Salt
- 100g smoked salmon
- Two boxes cress
- One bunch dill (20 g)
- Six eggs
- Pepper
- 4 tbsps. mineral water
- 4 tbsps. kefir (80 g)
- 4 tbsps. olive oil

Preparation
1. Wash the cucumber and cut diagonally into thin slices. Set aside some cucumber slices, lay out the rest on plates and sprinkle with salt.
2. Dice salmon. Cut cress from the beds. Wash dill, shake dry and chop.
3. Whisk eggs with salt, pepper, mineral water and kefir and stir in dill. Heat 3 spoons of oil inside a frying pan. Add half of the egg

combine and then cook over low heat in 3-4 minutes to an omelet. Roast a second omelet with the rest of the eggs.
4. Cover the omelets with salmon cubes, cucumber slices, and cress, fold them, cut in half and arrange on the cucumber slices.

Nutritional Information - Composition Amount (g) CDR (%)
Calories: 272

3. Chicken and leek salad

Preparation Time: 35 minutes

Ingredients for 4 portions
- 450g chicken breast fillet
- Salt
- Pepper
- 2 tbsps. olive oil
- 3 bars leek
- Two small apples (300 g)
- ½ lemons (juice)
- 50 ml of vegetable stock
- 2 tbsps. red wine vinegar
- 1 tsp. mustard
- 1 tsp. maple syrup
- 50g yogurt (3.5% fat)
- 1 tsp. paprika
- 1 tbsp. light sesame seeds (15 g)

Preparation
1. Rinse chicken breast fillets, pat dry and season with salt and pepper. Heat 1 tbsp. oil in a pan; roast the chicken meat for 4-5 minutes, turning it over. Then place in an ovenproof dish and cook in a preheated oven at 110 ° C (circulating air 90 ° C, gas: stage 1-2) in about 8-10 minutes.
2. Meanwhile, fresh leek, wash and cut diagonally into rings, heat 1 tbsp. oil in the pan. Brown leeks in medium heat for about 5 minutes, season with salt and pepper, remove from heat and let

cool for 5 minutes. While doing so, wash apples, quarter them, core them, cut them into thin slices and drizzle with lemon juice.
3. Whisk the vegetable stock, vinegar, salt, pepper, mustard, maple syrup and remaining oil and stir in the yogurt.
4. Take the roasted chicken from the oven and let it cool for 5 minutes. Mix the leek with the apple slices, spread on plates and drizzle with the dressing. Slice chicken breasts in slices and place on plates. Sprinkle chicken and leek salad with paprika and sesame seeds and serve.

Nutritional Information - Composition Amount (g) CDR (%)
Calories: 290 kcal

4. Italian bruschetta (several recipes)

The Italian bruschetta is a classic aperitif at all tables in the country, and there are many variations from the classic recipe we give you.

Ingredients
- Baguette homemade bread
- Ripe tomatoes 'Zwiebelart.'
- Fresh mozzarella
- Bold garlic
- Extra virgin olive oil
- Salt and fresh basil leaves

Preparations
1. Cut the bread into slices of about 2 cm. It can be baked or fried in the oven, in a traditional toaster or a coated pan with a peeling oil and raw garlic.
2. The tomatoes are washed, chopped and the seeds removed. You can drain into a flask to release the liquid.
3. Then season with salt and add chopped basil leaves and a drop of olive oil.
4. Cut the mozzarella into small cubes and add to the tomato mixture.
5. To collect the bruschettas, rub the toast with small raw garlic and cover it with tomato and cheese salad. They are currently being served.

Nutritional Information - Composition Amount (g) CDR (%)
Calories: 57.9
Monounsaturated Fat: 1.7 g
Dietary Fiber: 1 g
Sodium: 261.3mg

5. Zucchini carrots buffer

Preparation Time: 30 minutes
Thanks to plenty of vegetables, these buffers contain a lot of fiber and make you full for a long time. Carrots contain a series of beta-carotene, a precursor of vitamin A. The fat-soluble vitamin is vital for healthy eyes.

Ingredients for 4 portions
- 500g predominantly hard-boiling potatoes
- Two carrots
- One zucchini
- 1 tbsp. chickpea flour (15 g)
- salt
- nutmeg
- 2 tbsps. olive oil
- One organic lemon
- ½ bunch rocket (40 g)

Preparation
1. Peel potatoes. Wash carrots and zucchini and clean. Grate everything roughly and mix with the chickpea flour, season with salt and freshly grated nutmeg.
2. Heat olive oil inside a pan and add the potato mixture in portions. Press lightly flat and fry on medium heat from each side for about 6 minutes.
3. Meanwhile, wash the lemon hot, pat dry and cut into slices. Wash the rocket and then spin dry. Arrange buffers on 4 plates and then garnish with rocket. Lemon splits are enough.

Nutritional Information - Composition Amount (g) CDR (%)
Calories: 167 kcal

6. Rocket salad with mango, avocado and cherry tomatoes

Preparation Time: 15 minutes

Although avocados contain a lot of fat, because in addition to plenty of vitamin E score the green fruits with healthy polyunsaturated fatty acids, Mango has its yellow color due to the plant pigment beta carotene, which is a precursor of vitamin A, which is vital for healthy eyes. The cell-protecting lycopene from tomatoes completes the essential substance package.

Ingredients for 4 portions
- 1 tbsp. lime juice
- 2 tbsps. white balsamic vinegar
- 2 tbsps. rapeseed oil
- 2 tbsps. olive oil
- 1 tsp. honey
- 1 tsp. medium hot mustard
- Salt
- Pepper
- Three handful rocket (120 g)
- 200g cherry tomatoes
- One ripe mango
- Two avocados

Preparation
1. For the vinaigrette, whip lime juice with balsamic vinegar, rapeseed and olive oils. Whisk in honey and mustard and then season with salt and pepper.
2. Wash the rocket and spin dry. Wash tomatoes and halve. Peel the mango, slice the pulp from the core and dice it. Halve the avocados, core them, remove the pulp from the skin and dice them as well. Add cherry tomatoes, ripe mango, avocados - all the salad ingredients inside a bowl with the vinaigrette and spread on 4 plates.

Nutritional Information - Composition Amount (g) CDR (%)
Calories: 306 kcal

7. Steamed Cod

Preparation Time: 30 minutes

The high-quality protein in the cod stimulates the metabolism and serves as a building material for cells, muscles, enzymes, and hormones. Valuable proteins also prevent cravings and muscle breakdown.

Ingredients for 4 portions
- 4 cod fillets - fish fillets (à 150 g)
- 4 tbsps. lemon juice
- 2 bars leek
- 3 tbsps. rapeseed oil
- 100 ml of vegetable stock
- salt
- pepper
- ½ dried thyme
- ½ bunch chives (10 g)
- One organic lemon

Preparation
1. Rinse the cod fillets, pat dry and drizzle with 2 tbsps. lemon juice. Clean leeks, wash and cut into rings.
2. Heat 1 tbsps. rapeseed oil in a pan, dab fish dry, sauté for 2 minutes at medium heat. Then turn over, add the remaining lemon juice and 50 ml of vegetable stock and cover, cook for 5-7 minutes on low heat.
3. Meanwhile, heat remaining oil in a saucepan, sauté the leek rings in medium heat for 2 minutes, season with salt, pepper, and thyme. Add remaining vegetable stock and cook the leek for 5 minutes over low heat.
4. Meanwhile, wash chives, shake dry and cut into small rolls. Rinse lemon hot and cut into quarters
5. Season fish fillets and leeks with salt and pepper, arrange on plates and garnish with chives and lemon quarters.

Nutritional Information - Composition Amount (g) CDR (%)
Calories: 226 kcal

8. Quinoa and vegetable burger

Preparation Time: 25 minutes
Cooking Time: 10 minutes
Make this delicious quinoa burger with vegetables and vegan burger buns, which will be a sensation for people who value what they consume. It is very juicy and tasty.

<u>Ingredients</u> for 3 portions
- 1 cup cooked chickpea
- 2 tablespoons chia soaked in water
- 1/2 cup cooked quinoa
- 1/2 cup grated and pressed carrot
- 2 tablespoons sunflower seed
- 1/2 cup breadcrumbs
- 3 pinches of salt
- 1 pinch of pepper
- 1/2 cup coconut oil
- 1 piece of pepper cut into a leaf
- Cut 1 piece of pumpkin into thin slices
- 2 pinches of salt
- 1 pinch of pepper
- 1 piece avocado
- 1 tablespoon of lemon juice
- 2 pinches of salt
- 3 pieces of vegan burger bread

<u>Preparation</u>
1. Process the chickpeas inside a food processor for 3 minutes until you receive a puree.
2. In a bowl, mix the chickpea puree with chia, quinoa, carrots, sunflower seeds, breadcrumbs, salt, and pepper.
3. Form hamburger with the chickpea mixture and fry on low heat with a little coconut oil in a pan until they are cooked. Drain on absorbent paper and reserve.
4. In a bowl, mix the pepper, the pumpkin; add two tablespoons of coconut oil; Season and reserve.

5. In a bowl crush the avocado with the juice, lemon, and salt until you get a puree.
6. Heat the vegan hamburger buns, serve the burgers with pepper and pumpkin in the bread rolls, add the avocado puree and serve. Enjoy

Nutritional Information - Composition Amount (g) CDR (%) - Percent of daily values based on a 2,000-calorie diet
Calories: 1066 kcal, 53%
Carbohydrates: 117g, 39%
Proteins: 32.0g, 64%
Lipids: 55.0g, 85%
Fiber: 25.1g, 50%
Sugar: 13.8g, 15%
Cholesterol: 0.0mg, 0.0%

9. Quinoa and vegetable spring rolls

Preparation Time: 20 minutes
The recipe for quinoa and vegetable spring rolls is perfect for the youngest household members. It is a healthy and rich preparation, which makes the rolls an excellent option for lunch for your children.

Ingredients for 4 portions
- 1 rice paper
- 1/3 cup of quinoa
- 1/2 red pepper
- 1/2 cup of spinach
- 1/2 cup carrot
- 1/2 cucumber
- 1 teaspoon salt
- 1 pinch of pepper
- 1 cup of grape

Preparation
1. Soak the quinoa and drain the water.

2. Place the quinoa right inside a saucepan with 2/3 cup of water and a pinch of salt and add pepper and then bring to a boil over medium heat for 10 minutes with the pot closed.
3. While the quinoa is still cooking, cut the carrots, cucumbers, and peppers into thin sticks.
4. Place some water into a large bowl and let one of the rice papers soak for 20 seconds.
5. Insert the stretched rice paper and add quinoa, red peppers, carrots, cucumbers, and spinach.
6. Roll the rice paper with all the ingredients in it. Add grape, cut the roll into small pieces.

Nutritional Information - Percent of daily values based on a 2,000-calorie diet.
Calories: 152 kcal, 7.6%
Carbohydrates: 31.4g, 10%
Proteins: 5.1g, 10%
Lipids: 2.0g, 3.1%
Fiber: 4.0g, 7.9%
Sugar: 13.3g, 15%

10. Asparagus Soup with Salmon

Preparation Time: 30 minutes
Creamy asparagus soup of white asparagus with a delicious addition of smoked salmon

<u>Ingredients</u> for 6 people
- 700 gr asparagus
- 2 cubes of chicken broth
- 200 ml of cream
- 80 gr flour/cornflour
- 70 gr butter
- 150 gr smoked salmon
- 2 shallots
- Fresh chives
- Hand of croutons
- Fresh parsley to garnish

Preparation
1. Cut the asparagus into pieces. Boil for 5 minutes in about 1.5 liters of water and then cook for 10 minutes in the water. Finely chop the shallots. Dissolve the butter in a soup pan and fry the shallots in it. Then add the flour and stir with a whisk to a roux and let it bake and cook for 5 minutes. Drain the asparagus and collect all the cooking liquid.
2. Dissolve the bouillon cubes in the cooking liquid of the asparagus. Pour this little by little at the roux and keep stirring with a whisk so that no lumps arise. When all chicken broth has been added, stir in the cream and add croutons and the cooked asparagus.
3. Taste whether the soup is well-flavored and add a pinch of pepper and salt if necessary. Add the salmon (partially) in strips to the soup. Spoon the soup into plates and parsley garnish with salmon and some chopped chives.

Nutritional Information - Composition Amount (g) CDR (%)
Calories: 86.3
Total Fat: 3.2 g
Saturated Fat: 1.6 g
Polyunsaturated Fat: 0.4 g
Monounsaturated Fat: 0.9 g
Cholesterol: 8.4mg
Sodium: 927.1mg
Potassium: 259.2mg
Total Carbohydrate: 11.1 g
Dietary Fiber: 1.7 g
Sugars: 2.5 g
Protein: 4.6 g

11. Pasta salad with corn, avocado, and tomato

Preparation time: 20 minutes
Cooking time: 10 minutes
Total time: 30 minutes

Ingredients for 6 people
- 1 package of 450-500 grams of short pasta the one you prefer

- 1 pound of tender corn or shelled corn can be fresh, canned or frozen
- The juice of 1 large lemon
- 1 tablespoon Dijon-type mustard
- 4 tablespoons of olive oil
- 2 tomatoes (large), cut into cubes can also be replaced with cherry tomatoes
- 1/2 red onion, cut in cubes (wash them in cold water to remove the strong flavor)
- 2 tablespoons chopped cilantro - you can also use parsley /basil/dill
- 1 jalapeno or hot pepper, without seeds or veins, finely chopped - optional (you can substitute it with sweet pepper or omit if you do not want it spicy)
- 1-2 avocados, diced or sliced
- Salt and pepper to taste

Preparation
1. Cook the pasta according to package instructions. You can add the grains of tender corn during the last 4-5 minutes of cooking the pasta. If you are using Andean corn, the same one that needs more cooking time, you can cook it separately.
2. Drain the pasta and corn. Let it cool down a bit.
3. For the dressing, put lemon juice, Dijon-type mustard, olive oil, salt and pepper in a bowl or small jar. Mix well.
4. Put the pasta and corn in a large salad bowl. Add the chopped tomatoes, the chopped red onions (and washed in cold water), the sweet pepper or the chili / chopped chili, and the chopped cilantro.
5. Place the dressing to the salad and then mix well.
6. If it is going to be served immediately, add the avocado. Otherwise, you can save the salad in the refrigerator and add the avocado just before serving.

Nutritional Information - Composition Amount (g) CDR (%)
Calories: 90.2
Total Fat: 4.6g
Dietary Fiber: 2.5g
Saturated Fat: 1.7g

12. Layered salad of crab with avocado

Preparation time: 20 minutes
Recipe for a delicious and easy salad of layers of crab and avocado, this salad is prepared with a layer of avocado covered with a layer of fresh crab salad mixed with red onion, pepper, cucumber, radishes, lemon juice, olive oil, and cilantro.

Ingredients for 4 people
For the crab salad layer
- ½ pound of cooked crab meat, reserve some pieces to add on top
- ¼ red onion, finely chopped
- ¼ red pepper, finely chopped
- ½ green pepper, finely chopped
- ¼ cucumber, finely chopped
- 2-3 radishes, finely chopped
- 1-2 tablespoons of finely chopped cilantro
- Juice of 2 small lemons or use 1 large lemon
- 2 tablespoons of olive oil
- Salt and pepper to taste

For the avocado salad layer
- 2 large ripe avocados
- 1-2 tablespoons of lemon juice
- Olive oil to taste
- Salt to taste

Additional fittings
- Pickled onions
- Coriander leaves, parsley, etc.

Preparation
For the crab salad layer
1. In a bowl or large bowl, combine the cooked crab meat with chopped onions, chopped peppers, diced cucumbers, chopped radish, and cilantro. Mix well.
2. Add lemon juice, olive oil and little salt/pepper to taste.

3. The salad can also be prepared in advance and then kept refrigerated until ready to serve and assemble the layers of avocado and crab.

For the avocado salad layer
4. Peel and chop the avocados in squares. Sprinkle with lemon juice, olive oil, and salt to taste. The avocado can be cut into cubes, into thin slices or crushed and pureed for a creamier texture.
5. To assemble and serve the layers of crab and avocado salad:
6. Place a lightly greased round pan with a little oil in the center of each dish, add the chopped or crushed avocado layer first, press gently down (using a spoon) to enable it as compact as possible.
7. Then, add a generous layer of the crab salad. Press down and then gently remove the mold.
8. If you kept some pieces of crab, add them to the top. You can also decorate the salad with coriander leaves and pickled red onions.

Notes
For a complete layer salad, you can add a layer of rice to cilantro as the first layer. For a spicy variation, add chopped jalapeños or other hot peppers/peppers to the avocado layer.

Nutritional Information - Composition Amount (g) CDR (%)
Calories: 445.1
Saturated Fat: 5.8 g
Total Fat: 5.8 g
Polyunsaturated Fat: 2.8 g

13. Salad of palm heart, jicama, and avocado (Tropical mixed salad)

Preparation time: 30 minutes
This refreshing mixed salad of heart of palm, jicama, and avocado is prepared with lettuce, hearts of palm, jicama, avocado, orange, cucumber, radish, onion, and has an avocado and cilantro dressing.

Ingredients for 6 people
For avocado and lemon and cilantro dressing
- 1 small ripe avocado
- 1 bunch of coriander leaves adjusted to your liking

- ¼ cup of lemon juice of about 2 lemons
- 1 to 2 jalapeños or hot peppers/chili peppers without seeds/veins (use sweet green pepper or paprika if desired without spicy) - adjust to your liking
- Salt to taste

For the mixed salad of palmito, avocado
- 8 ounces of lettuce leaves or a mixture of lettuce, spinach, arugula, etc.
- 6 palm hearts ~ 9 ounces, cut into slices
- ½ small of jicama peeled and then cut into thin strips
- 1 large ripe but firm avocado, peeled, boneless, and diced
- 2 peeled and sliced oranges in supreme style
- 4 radishes cut into thin slices
- ½ cucumber cut into thin slices
- ½ red onion cut into thin slices and washed in cold water

Additional side dishes (optional) for the salad
- Tortilla chips
- Cheese crumbled strawberries can also use feta cheese or the one you want
- Coriander leaves

Preparation
For the dressing
1. Put all the ingredients inside a blender or a mini-food processor and blend well until you get a creamy dressing. Taste and then adjust the taste to your liking.

For the mixed salad
2. The salad can be prepared in a long bowl or a bowl for salads.
3. To serve it at the source, place the lettuce leaves first in the dish, covering the entire surface. Then add each vegetable or fruit as if you were making a rainbow.
4. To serve it in a bowl, add the lettuce leaves and spread the rest of the chopped vegetables/fruits on top.

5. Add lemon juice, the avocado dressing when serving the salad, along with the additional side dishes (tortilla chips, shredded cheese, and coriander leaves).

Nutritional Information - Composition Amount (g) CDR (%)
Total Fat: 5g, 7%
Sugar: 1g, 1%
Fatty acids, total saturated: 4g, 17%
Cholesterol: 4mg, 1%
Protein: 2g, 4%
Carbohydrate, by difference: 2g, 2%

14. Light Mushroom Risotto

Preparation time: 35 minutes
It is a recipe super nutritious and very easy to prepare, which can bring us a lot of energy.

Ingredients
- Five medium potatoes
- 300g of mushrooms
- 250g of arborous rice or carnaroli
- One onion
- One clove garlic
- 1 l of vegetable broth
- One glass of white wine
- 50g of Parmesan cheese
- 4 tablespoons of olive oil
- A sprig of parsley
- Salt and pepper

Preparation
1. Heat the vegetable broth. Put the vegetable broth to heat. Wash the parsley, potatoes, dry it, reserve some whole leaves for decorating and chopping the rest. Grate the Parmesan cheese.
2. Poach the garlic and onion. Peel and clean the garlic and onion, and chop them. In a casserole with olive oil, beat them for about 5 minutes or so over low heat.

3. Skip the mushrooms. Meanwhile, clean the mushrooms. Leave a few whole pieces for decoration and the rest of the pieces in small pieces. Add them all to the casserole and sauté everything around five more minutes.
4. Incorporate the rice. Once you have sautéed the mushrooms with the onion and garlic, remove the ones that you had left whole and reserve them. Add the rice to the pan, arborous rice or carnaroli and then sauté everything together for another 5 minutes, stirring constantly.
5. Make the risotto. Pour the glass of white wine and a broth of broth, and cook for 15 minutes, stirring frequently, and adding broth as the rice absorbs it.
6. Complete the risotto. After the indicated time, add the cheese, parsley, salt and pepper to taste, and the rest of the broth and cook for three more minutes, stirring vigorously. Let stand 2 minutes, and serve.

Nutritional Information - Composition Amount (g) CDR (%)
Calories: 111
Total Fat: 2 g
Carbohydrates: 19 g
Fiber: 0 g
Sugar: 18 g
Calcium: 15%
Iron: 0%

15. Light Lentil Stew

It is a highly versatile recipe because you can make it to your liking; that means putting the vegetables you like the most and making them as colorful as you like a pleasure you can enjoy.
Preparation time: 1 hour
Ingredients
- 250g of brownish lentils
- One zucchini
- Two carrots
- One onion
- One clove garlic

- One bay leaf
- Two small branch tomatoes
- One piece of ginger (optional)
- Three teaspoons of olive oil
- Two sprigs of coriander or parsley
- Salt and pepper

Preparation
1. Prepare the vegetables. First, peel the onion and the garlic, and chop them. Then, peel the ginger, and chop it too fine. And finally, peel the carrot, wash the zucchini, remove them, and cut them into cubes.
2. Sauté the vegetables. Heat 2 teaspoons of oil in a casserole, add half of the onion and garlic and cook for 3 or 4 minutes or so. Then add the ginger, bay leaf, carrot, and zucchini, and sauté a little.
3. Cook the lentils. After sautéing the vegetables, add the lentils. Cover with 3/4 of a liter (750 ml) of water, and cook over low heat for 45 minutes till the lentils are tender, and reserve.
4. Assemble the plate.
5. Finally, wash the tomatoes and chop them. Mix them with the rest of the onion and garlic, and season them with salt, pepper and the remaining oil. Divide the lentils into 4 bowls or bowls, and add the tomato hash and some leaves of coriander or parsley.
6. And if you want a fresh and ultra-fast version, instead of stewing the lentils, you can buy them already cooked and make a salad. You have to sauté the vegetables a little, but not too much so that they remain al dente. And mix them with the lentils already cooked and drained, and the tomato hash.

Nutritional Information - Composition Amount (g) CDR (%)
Calories: 111
Total Fat: 2g
Saturated Fat: 1g
Cholesterol: 10mg
Sodium: 58mg
Carbohydrates: 19g
Fiber: 0 g
Sugar: 18 g
Calcium: 15%

Iron: 0%

16. Salad of red beans with guacamole

Preparation time: 30 minutes
Ingredients for 4 people
- 1 unit (s) of Tomato (medium)
- 1 unit (s) of Onion (half onion purple)
- 1 unit (s) of red pepper (medium)
- 1 pinch of Pepper
- 1 unit (s) of Limón
- 1 pinch of salt
- 1 unit (s) of Green pepper
- 250 grams of Azuki a pot (canned red beans already cooked)
- 1 tablespoon of extra virgin olive oil
- 1 unit (s) of fresh Guacamole Frutas Montosa (Mercadona) but you can make it homemade too
- 1 small cup of sweet corn in a can

Preparation
1. Prepare the salad by mixing all the chopped ingredients with the beans previously washed and drained.
2. Dress with lemon juice and oil and season with salt and pepper.
3. Serve the salad with the guacamole and toast with toasted bread.

Nutritional Information - Composition Amount (g) CDR (%)
Composition Amount (gr) CDR (%)
Calories: 353.04, 18.4%
Carbohydrates: 42.06g, 13.5%
Proteins: 14.75g, 30.8%
Fiber: 13.82g, 46.1%
Fat: 10.33g, 19.4%

17. Salad with avocado and black beans

This time we bring you a recipe of avocado salad (with diced beans) super nutritious that you will love. The avocado has become, by its own merits, an indispensable Ingredients in our pantry. Not only is it very nutritious and contains all kinds of healthy fats for our body or vitamin E for your skin, it also gives a lot of creaminess and flavor to your recipes, being a perfect substitute for oil or ideal for preparing your creamy 100% vegetable sauces.

Preparation time: 10 minutes

Ingredients for 3 people
- 2 unit (s) of Tomato
- 1 unit (s) of Avocado
- 1 pinch of Cilantro
- 1 unit (s) of Cebolleta (green onion)
- 1 pinch of Modena balsamic vinegar
- 1 pinch of lemon juice
- 1 pinch of extra virgin olive oil
- 1.5 glass of canned red beans

Preparation
1. Divide the avocado and tomato into cubes and the spring onion into thin slices and place it in a salad bowl.
2. We add the beans and mix well.
3. Prepare vinaigrette with lemon juice, vinegar, oil, and salt, and sprinkle it on top.
4. We put a little cilantro to taste and mix everything.

Note
Can be used as fajitas filling too, it is delicious!

Nutritional Information - Composition Amount (g) CDR (%)
Calories: 204.77, 10.7%
Carbohydrates: 19.38g, 6.2%
Proteins: 9g, 18.8%
Fiber: 7.58g, 25.3%
Fat: 8.59g, 16.2%

18. Green smoothie with oats

Preparation time: 5 minutes

Ingredients for 1 person
- 1 pinch of spinach 5 or 6 leaves, to taste
- 0.5 unit (s) of Cucumber
- 0.5 unit (s) of Apple
- 1 unit (s) of Pineapple fresh slice
- 3 tablespoon of Oats
- 1 glass of water
- 4 grams of Ginger
- 1 tablespoon of Flaxseeds

Preparation
1. Wash and split the fruits and vegetables and place them in the beater, ginger, apple and cucumber with skin.
2. Oatmeal, linen and a stream of cold water are added to the taste so that it is higher or less thick according to the taste of each one.
3. Ready for breakfast or snacks. It helps clean and fills a lot.

Nutritional Information - Composition Amount (gr) CDR (%)
Calories: 645.68, 33.7%
Carbohydrates: 106.08g, 34.1%
Proteins: 13.96g, 29.2%
Fiber: 23.71g, 79%
Fat: 15.32g, 28.8%
Calcium: 193.99mg, 16.2%
Iron: 8.15mg, 101.9%
Magnesium: 245.14mg, 58.4%
Match: 415.61mg, 59.4%
Potassium: 1510.44mg, 75.5%

19. Detoxifying milkshake

Preparation time: 10 minutes

Ingredients for 2 people
- 1 cup of Celery (one head)
- 2 glass of Spinach
- 2 glass of Cucumber
- 1 unit (s) of Limón
- 2 unit (s) of Apple
- 1 pinch of fresh ginger

Preparation
Put all the ingredients together inside the blender and blend until a homogeneous mixture is obtained.

Nutritional Information - Composition Amount (gr) CDR (%)
Calories: 191.21, 10%
Carbohydrates: 29.52g, 9.5%
Proteins: 7.32g, 15.3%
Fiber: 13.69g, 45.6%
Fat: 1.88g, 3.5%
Sodium: 158.44mg, 9.9%
Calcium: 273.33mg, 22.8%
Iron: 6.82mg, 85.3%
Magnesium: 156.7mg, 37.3%
Match: 163.19mg, 23.3%
Potassium: 1691.3mg, 84.6%
Vitamin A: 1.16mg, 129.1%
Vitamin B1: 0.36mg, 30%
Vitamin B2: 0.51mg, 39%
Vitamin B3: 3.75mg, 0%
Vitamin C: 148.16mg, 164.6%

20. Green pineapple smoothie

Preparation time: 5 minutes

Ingredients for 1 person
- 50 grams of Chard
- 1 unit (s) of Apple
- 200 grams of Pineapple
- 1 teaspoon of Flaxseeds

Preparation
All to the glass of the blender with a little water and grind well.

Nutritional Information - Composition Amount (gr) CDR (%)
Calories: 251.16, 13.1
Carbohydrates: 46.44g, 14.9%
Proteins: 3.51g, 7.3%
Fiber: 9.88g, 32.9%
Fat: 4.11g, 7.7%
Sodium: 83.28mg, 5.2%
Calcium: 107.25mg, 8.9%
Iron: 3.88mg, 48.5%
Magnesium: 100.44mg, 23.9%
Match: 99.42mg, 14.2%
Potassium: 816.78mg, 40.8%
Vitamin A: 0.19mg, 20.6%
Vitamin B1: 0.36mg, 30%
Vitamin B2: 0.15mg, 11.7%
Vitamin B3: 1.74mg, 0%
Vitamin C: 63.03mg, 70%

21. Baby spinach, chicken and carrot salad with red wine dressing

Ingredients
- Carrots: 2
- Red onions: 3

- Spinach sprouts: 80 g
- Olive oil: 3 tbsp. soup
- Lemon juice: 0.5 tbsp. coffee
- Juice of 1/2 orange
- Agave syrup: 1 tbsp. coffee

Preparation
1. Peel the carrots and onions. Cut the carrots into slices using a thrifty knife and sliced onions.
2. Wash the spinach sprouts, and then drain them. Mix in a medium bowl with the carrots and onions.
3. Mix the agave syrup with the olive oil and the orange and lemon juice. Pour over the salad and mix before serving. Enjoy it immediately.

22. Chicken and Bacon Salad

All these flavors together taste great: chicken, bacon, lettuce, tomato... It's a great combination, but why leaves it there? Make this delicious salad something even more keto by adding a good dose of creamy aioli.

Ingredients
- 450g boneless chicken thighs
- 30g butter
- 225g bacon
- 110g cherry tomatoes
- 275g romaine lettuce
- Salt and ground black pepper
- Aioli
- 175 ml (150 g) mayonnaise
- ½ tbsp garlic powder

Preparation
1. Mix the mayonnaise and garlic powder in a small bowl and set aside.

2. Fry the bacon slices in butter until they are crispy. Remove them from the pan and then keep them warm. Store the accumulated fat in the pan.
3. Crumble the chicken and salt and pepper. Fry inside the same pan as the chicken until golden brown and fully cooked.
4. Rinse the lettuce and cut it into strips. Be sure to use a different cutting board than the one you used for chicken. Put the lettuce on a plate together with the chicken, bacon, tomatoes and a good dose of garlic mayonnaise.

Nutritional Information - Composition Amount (g) CDR (%) per portion
Calories: 836
Fat: 78g, 85%
Fiber: 2 g
Protein: 28g, 13%

23. Pumpkin and apple soup

Ingredients
- 450 grams (1 lb.) pumpkin
- 1 Granny Smith apple cored, and quartered
- One medium onion cut
- Two cloves garlic
- One tablespoon of olive oil
- salt
- ¼ teaspoon of cayenne more to taste
- 300 ml (1¼ cup) of vegetable stock
- freshly ground black pepper to add taste

Garnish

- pomegranate arils
- some pumpkin seeds
- fresh parsley finely chopped

Preparation
1. Preheat the oven about 200 degrees C (or 392 degrees F). Line a large baking sheet with a parchment paper.

2. Cut the pumpkin half lengthways and scoop out seeds.
3. Slice each pumpkin half in half to make quarters and place, cut-side up, on a baking tray, along with the onions.
4. Drizzle with olive oil and then sprinkle some salt.
5. Bake for about 20 minutes, then add the garlic and apple, flip the pumpkin cut side down and then roast for another for 20 minutes, or until the flesh is soft.
6. Use a spoon to scoop out the flesh of the pumpkin and transfer to a high-speed blender with the apple, onion, garlic (remove the skins), cayenne, and vegetable stock.
7. Blend on high for almost 2 minutes, or until silky smooth.
8. If too thick, add vegetable stock to thin it out and blend over. Taste and adjust the seasonings.
9. Serve, ladle soup into a bowl, and with pomegranate arils, pumpkin seeds, fresh parsley and freshly ground black pepper.
10. Then serve.
11. Refrigerate leftovers inside an airtight container for 4 days.

24. Reds salad on bacon and balsamic vinaigrette

Ingredients
- Balsamic vinaigrette:
- ¼ cup olive oil
- Three tablespoons balsamic vinegar
- ½ teaspoon finely chopped garlic
- ¾ Dijon mustard spoon
- ¾ honey bee teaspoon
- Salt and pepper to taste
- Salad with red grapes, bacon, and walnut:
- 3 cups mixed lettuce (escarole, French, ball, Italian)
- ½ cup red grapes, in halves
- Two slices of bacon, golden brown
- 8-10 praline or natural walnuts
- Two tablespoons blue cheese, Roquefort or blue cheese

Preparation

1. Balsamic vinegar vinaigrette:
2. Mix all ingredients in a jar, cup or dish and mix well until everything is well incorporated.
3. Add season to taste.
4. Salad with red grapes:
5. Cook the bacon until well browned and cut into medium pieces.
6. Mix the lettuce with half of the balsamic vinaigrette.
7. Place on a plate.
8. Add the red grapes in halves, the bacon in pieces, the blue cheese, and the nuts.
9. Serve with the remaining vinaigrette.

25. Arugula, lettuce and strawberry salad

Ingredients
- ¼ red onion, thinly sliced
- 4 cups of arugula leaves
- 250g tapered strawberries
- 90g goat cheese crumbled
- 1 to 2 cases of balsamic vinegar
- 2 to 3 cases of olive oil
- The salt according to your taste

Preparation
1. Dip the onions in cold, lightly salted water to remove the bitter side.
2. Mix the balsamic vinegar, olive oil and salt in a tight container and shake to the rhythm of the salsa.
3. Drain the onions and mix with the arugula leaves and the vinaigrette.
4. Top with crumbled cheese, sliced strawberries, and spicy pecans.
5. Mix at the table and serve immediately.

26. Curry tuna salad

Ingredients
- 400g natural tuna one beautiful romaine 100g raisins two medium pippin apples one lemon juice one teaspoon curry 1 cup mayonnaise

Preparation
1. Open the can of tuna. Drain and divide into large pieces.
2. Wash and dry the salad leaves thoroughly. Peel apples before cutting into thin slices sprinkle the lemon juice to prevent them from turning black.
3. Dressing the tuna salad with curry:
4. In a salad bowl, arrange the salad leaves, the pieces of tuna, the raisins and the slices of apple to mix everything.
5. Add the curry to the mayonnaise and stir well.
6. Mix the mayonnaise with the salad just before serving.

27. Roasted carrots and cashew salad on lemon vinaigrette

Ingredients for 2 people
- 4 beautiful carrots
- One wrist of cashew nuts
- One wrist of parsley or coriander
- One tablespoon soup grape dry
- For seasoning:
- One lemon
- One tablespoon of tahini
- Two tablespoons of olive oil
- One tablespoon of hazelnut oil

Preparation
1. Peel the carrots and grate them. Put them on a serving plate. Mince the parsley and add to the carrots. Add the raisins on top.
2. Heat 1 tablespoon of vegetable oil in a skillet over high heat and sauté the cashews. Stir frequently, so they do not burn. When they

turn a beautiful golden color, place them on paper towels and salt them. Let it cool before adding them to the carrots.
3. Prepare the seasoning: squeeze the lemon and place the juice in a bowl. Add the tablespoon tahini and mix well with a fork to fully dilute the sesame puree. Add two tablespoons of olive oil including a tablespoon of hazelnut oil. Mix the sauce well to incorporate the oils.

CHAPTER 8: Breakfast recipes

28. Tomato, cheese and black olives salad recipe

Ingredients
- 3 ripe but firm tomatoes
- 125 grams of mozzarella cheese pearls
- 50 grams of black olives without bone
- 1 can of mackerel in oil
- 50 grams pickled pickles
- 50 grams of pickled onions
- 1 handful of croutons
- 1 jet of extra virgin olive oil
- 1 pinch of dried basil
- 1 pinch of salt

Preparation
1. To prepare our tomato salad and mozzarella cheese, we start washing and drying the tomatoes well. We chopped them and put them in a bowl.
2. Drain the olives and onions and put them with tomatoes. Drain the pickles, chop them and add them to the salad bowl. Drain the mackerel oil, crumble it into large pieces and add it.
3. Dress with oil, salt, and dried basil (if you have fresh better), stir well, and before serving to add the mozzarella pearls and croutons so that the bread does not become soft. Bon Appetite!
4. If you like this tomato salad, cheese, and black olives, and you want to continue cooking in my blog Cuca's sweet secrets await many more ideas.

29. Sweet Potato and Quinoa Croquettes

Ingredients
- 475g sweet potato
- 1.25 cooked quinoa

- 1/4 cup dried cranberries
- 1/8 cup chopped mint
- 2 chopped jalapeños (seeded)

Preparations
1. Spray a pan with coconut oil, cook the sweet potatoes, and once done, remove from heat.
2. Puree with cooked potatoes
3. Add cooked quinoa, jalapeños, mint and dried cranberries
4. Form small croquettes by hand and cook pan for 20 minutes over medium heat
5. Enjoy!

30. Cheese and avocado omelette

For brunch or as a snack, serve this Pingo Doce and avocado lactose-free cheese omelette. A simple, healthy, and delicious recipe.

Ingredients
- 4 eggs M
- 1 c. salt tea
- what chilli
- 1 c. olive oil soup
- 100g lactose-free fresh cheese Pingo Doce Pura Vida
- 50g watercress
- 1 avocado
- 1 diced beet

Preparation
1. In a bowl, beat eggs and season with salt and pepper.
2. Heat the oil in a non-stick frying pan, pour the eggs into the frying pan, simmer and slowly release the sides. Turn and cook for another 1 minute.
3. Remove to a serving plate.
4. Spread the cheese on one side of the omelette, put a layer of watercress, then the sliced avocado, and then the diced beets.
5. Close the omelette and serve immediately.

31. Chocolate Coconut Porridge

Ingredients
- 2 tablespoons cornstarch
- 2 tablespoons of grated coconut
- 4 glasses of milk
- 2 large spoons of chocolate powder

Preparation
1. First, put the milk and 2 tablespoons cornstarch.
2. Bring to the heat and add the well-grated coconut.
3. Finally, put the chocolate.
4. Stir until desired consistency.

32. Broccoli and pumpkin gratin

Broccoli and squash are two nutritious foods that we should include in our usual diet. In addition, they have a characteristic flavour that can be combined to obtain different and simply delicious dishes.
Combining it with pumpkin is, without a doubt, a success with which not only to enhance its benefits but its flavour. Both have few calories, and the squash provides vitamin C and components that are converted into vitamin A in our leather. On the other hand, it has been pointed out that pumpkin could have an antidiabetic effect. However, it is necessary that human studies be carried out to obtain conclusive data.

Ingredients
- 100 grams of broccoli
- 100 grams of pumpkin
- 50 grams of whole wheat bread.
- 2 tablespoons your oat milk.
- Grated cheese for gratin (to taste).
- Salt and pepper.
- Lemon zest.

Preparation

1. First, we must cut the pumpkin and broccoli into small pieces. Then, we will wash them well and steam them with little water. Wait until they are done (they do not need to be very soft).
2. Next, we choose the source where we go to gratin. We will put the vegetable in the bottom with a little salt and pepper, along with a little lemon zest. We will also add the bread pieces soaked in oat milk, and cheese to taste. Finally, we will take it to the oven to gratin.

33. Sauteed oriental

Ingredients
- 1 small broccoli
- Half medium pumpkin.
- 1/2 cup of almonds (we will soak them the night before).
- 1/2 teaspoon cumin
- 1 teaspoon turmeric.
- Chilli pepper crushed to taste.
- Juice of half a lemon.
- 3 tablespoons olive oil.
- 1/2 teaspoon coriander

Preparation
1. To start, we cut broccoli and squash into small pieces.
2. Now, we will prepare the dressing with the cumin, the oil, the lemon juice, the chilli, and the cilantro. We will mix everything well.
3. Then, in a large skillet, and with a little oil, sauté the broccoli, pumpkin, and almonds. Remember that the pieces of pumpkin and broccoli should be small to be done well. Add the chilli, if you wish.
4. After this, we will add the seasoning to the pumpkin, broccoli, and almonds.
5. Finally, continue cooking all the vegetables until they are tender and ready. The mixture is very tasty. Serve it in two dishes and accompany it with soy sauce, if it is to your liking.

34. Pumpkin and broccoli pudding

Ingredients
- A small broccoli
- A tender onion
- An apple.
- 300 grams of pumpkin
- 3 eggs.
- 2 tablespoons olive oil
- 1 tablespoon of flour.
- 1 dash of skim milk
- Salt, parsley, and pepper.

Preparation
1. We will start steaming broccoli. After this, we must grate the pumpkin to very thin strips and cut the apple into thin slices
2. Once this is done, we must preheat the oven to 200 degrees.
3. Now, in a pan and with oil, we will sauté the finely chopped onion, just like parsley.
4. In a bowl, we will beat the eggs until they are foamy, then introduce the broccoli in corsages, the grated pumpkin, the onion sauteed in oil, as well as the cut apple.
5. After this, we will season and add a dash of skim milk mixed previously with the flour.
6. We will take a tray or the mould that we want for the oven (this will be the final form of the pudding), and we will spread it on butter. Then, we must pour the mixture of all the previous ingredients.
7. We will introduce it in the oven for 20 or 25 minutes. We let cool and finally, we will unmold. You can accompany this tasty pudding with a vinaigrette.

35. Blueberry Smoothie I Blueberry Smoothie

Breakfast is one of the essential times to include nutrient-rich foods and antioxidants! And no doubt, a smoothie is one of the most practical ways to combine all of these ingredients into one preparation.

Blueberry is one of the most antioxidant fruits, and including fat in the recipe helps even more in absorbing these nutrients and regulating the blood glucose in the method! So, go for it! Here you will find some ingredients that I usually include in my recipes and their main benefits.

Ingredients (organic)
- 1 cup frozen blueberry
- 1/2 cup frozen cauliflower
- 1 cup almond milk
- 1/3 scoop of vegetable protein (use this one or this one)
- 1 teaspoon cinnamon
- 1 hand frozen raw spinach
- Fresh Ginger Chips
- 1 teaspoon vanilla without alcohol.
- 1 tsp Peruvian Maca (good adaptogenic for hormonal balance)
- 1 tsp reishi mushroom (strengthens the immune system)

Toppings: Coconut flakes, almond paste, and granola.
Preparation
1. Blend all ingredients until smooth and creamy in texture.
2. Add the toppings of your choice and enjoy!

36. Orange Salad with Olive Oil

Ingredients
- 1 good quality orange per person
- 1 ripe grenade (optional)
- Sugar
- Cinnamon
- Extra Virgin Olive Oil

Preparation
1. The first of the breakfast salads! We cut the ends of the orange in the opposite direction to the needles of the rejol, cutting the whole peel, including the white part.

2. Once the oranges are peeled, we cut them into wedges on top of the plate in which we are going to serve the salad so that the juice stays below.
3. Add the white sugar, cinnamon, arrange the pomegranate grains (optional), and water the dish with an extra virgin olive oil.

37. Sweet and Sour Papaya Salad

Ingredients
- 1/4 of fresh Papaya
- Tender leaf sprouts
- 6-8 sweet and sour pickles
- 2 tablespoons extra virgin olive oil
- Salt

Preparation
1. Peel the papaya, remove the seeds and chop it into thin slices, about 5 mm thick. We place the tender shoots and the papaya in the centre.
2. Prepare the dressing; for this, we will cut the very small pickles, mix them with the oil and salt, stir it well. Then we add it to papaya, and that's it! Have you seen how simple it is to make one of the salads for breakfast?

38. Jamaican Salad

Ingredients
- 2 bananas
- Lemon juice
- 2 oranges
- 1 grapefruit
- 200 gr. of cherries
- 30 gr. of hazelnuts
- 1/2 cup melon chips (balls or cubes)
- 2 chopped kiwis
- 100 gr. of mayonnaise
- 2 tablespoons of cream

- 1 tablespoon brandy
- Salt (optional)

Preparation
1. We wash the bananas with the peel. Then we cut in half and remove the pulp. We add the cherries.
2. Roast the nuts in a pan without using oil or butter.
3. After 10 minutes, remove the hazelnut skin by gently removing it with a towel. Crush the hazelnuts.
4. Mix mayonnaise, brandy, and lemon juice, adding a little salt.

39. Watermelon salad

This watermelon salad is not only full of delicious flavours and textures that will fascinate you. It is full of a thousand and one nutrients.

Ingredients
- 6 cups of watermelon
- 1/4 sliced purple onion as thin as you can
- 1 serrano chilli in super thin slices
- 1/4 basil chopped into strips
- 2 tablespoons lemon juice
- 4 tablespoons olive oil
- 1/2 teaspoon sea salt
- 1/2 cup chopped almonds

Preparation
1. Mix the almonds with the oil and a pinch of salt and put them in the toaster oven, in the oven or a little pan to brown. About 5-7 min. It depends on where you put them. They are ready when they start to smell good.
2. In a small bowl, mix the lemon juice and olive oil, season with salt.
3. In a large bowl, mix the watermelon (being careful not to mistreat it much), with basil, serrano pepper, onion.
4. Put the lemon and olive oil. Serve and finish it with the chopped almonds and a pinch of salt.

40. Avocado, Cucumber and Tomato Salad

Ingredients
- 1 cucumber
- 4 tomatoes
- 3 avocados
- ½ lilac onion
- ¼ cup chopped cilantro
- 1 lemon
- 2 tbsp extra virgin olive oil
- Salt to taste
- Pepper to taste

Preparation
1. Cut the cucumber, tomatoes, avocados, and lilac onion into pieces.
2. Incorporate them all in a bowl.
3. Add the cilantro.
4. Squeeze the lemon into the bowl.
5. Add the coriander, salt, and pepper.
6. Move it well.

41. Basil Tomato Mix

Ingredients
- 6 finely chopped scallions
- one purple onion chopped in brunoise
- 3 teeth crushed the garlic
- 1 handful tightly packed fresh basil leaves finely chopped
- 300 gr Ground beef
- 1 level scoop dehydrated basil
- 1 tablespoon oregano
- 1/2 black pepper blade
- one sea salt knife
- 4-5 chopped ripe, ripe tomatoes concassé
- 2 envelopes Italian tomato sauce
- 1 jet frying oil

- 2 leaves laurel

Preparation
1. Fry together the chives and purple onion add garlic and fresh basil. Mix well. Add the meat.
2. Chop the tomatoes and add them to our mixture, mix well and add the bay leaves.
3. Add the tomato sauce, the two envelopes, one at a time. Mix and add sea salt.
4. Add the dried basil and pepper — also, oregano.
5. Mix well stir, correct seasoning and add some boiled water. Serve immediately on the pasta of your choice.

42. Green Corn Salad with Tomato

This salad is prepared with fresh oregano, mint and cilantro, and spinach leaves, but don't get caught up in it. Use your favorite herbs and leaves or those within reach. The sauce has cumin powder as its main Ingredients, which, despite its strong flavor, does not stand out from the mild flavor of corn.

Ingredients
Salad:
- 2 ½ cups (280 g) fresh green corn kernels
- 10 to 12 small ripe and firm tomatoes
- 1 small peeled cucumber, seedless, diced
- 1 small onion, red or white, diced
- ½ cup fresh minced herbs (oregano, mint, coriander, basil, dill, etc.)
- Salt and freshly ground black pepper to taste
- 3-4 cups fresh spinach or other favourite green leaves, well washed and drained

Sauce:
- 1 teaspoon ground cumin
- 1 clove minced or mashed garlic
- 2 tbsp red wine vinegar or balsamic vinegar
- ⅓ cup (75 ml) olive oil

Preparation
1. Salad: In a large bowl, put the corn, tomatoes - cut in half the large ones - cucumber, onion, and fresh herbs; set it aside.
2. Sauce: Heat a small skillet over moderate heat and add the cumin. Let it toast, constantly stirring, for about 20 seconds or until the aroma is released and begins to change colour. Transfer it to a small bowl; add garlic, vinegar and mix well with a fork or hand whisk. Gradually add the olive oil, always beating until a homogeneous sauce is formed. Pour it over the salad and mix well. Season with salt and pepper cover and let stand at room temperature for 20 to 30 minutes.
3. Assembly: Add the spinach leaves and mix gently. Transfer to a salad bowl, garnish to taste and serve.
4. Serves 4 to 6 servings
5. Suggestion: Try serving this salad at room temperature. If you need to refrigerate it, let it return to room temperature, and add the spinach leaves just before serving.

43. Italian Muffins

Ingredients
- Ragú tomato sauce
- Bolillo or Telera bread
- Black olives
- Onion
- Cold meat of your choice
- Mozzarella cheese
- Spinach

Preparation
1. You open the bread and remove the crumb, with a teaspoon spread the tomato sauce, add the cold meats (pepperoni, ham, Winny, bacon) whatever you have in the fridge, you can make them Hawaiian with ham and pineapple. You also add the sliced black olives, spinach, and in the end the grated cheese.
2. Put all the muffins in a tray and bake until the cheese is au gratin.

44. Carrot And Coconut Muffins For Breakfast

Ingredients
- 2 cups of flour
- 4 carrots
- Chemical yeast
- Baking soda
- 1 cup of brown sugar
- 1.5 dl of milk
- 1 egg
- Butter
- 1/2 cup shredded coconut
- Salt

Preparation
1. Preheat the oven to 180° C: wash and grate the carrots. Beat the egg and a cup of brown sugar in a bowl. When the eggs foam, add 1.5 dl of milk and the finely grated carrot. Mix everything well.
2. Sift 2 cups of flour, a teaspoon of yeast, and 1/2 de bicarbonate over the mixture. Add a teaspoon of salt and mix everything with enveloping movements so that the dough is aerated and thin.
3. Butter the muffin moulds. Spread the mixture in the molds and sprinkle grated coconut on top. Bake in preheated oven and bake about 20 minutes until the muffins rise and brown.

45. Raw Zucchini Salad with Feta

Ingredients for 4 people
- 2 large zucchini cut into thin slices
- 200g feta cheese
- 4 hard-boiled eggs
- 2 large onions and 4 tomatoes cut into pieces
- black olives
- basil, salt, pepper
- vinaigrette

Preparation
1. Remove the zucchini by placing them in a colander with coarse salt for 1/2 hour.
2. In the meantime, cook the eggs, slice them, cut them into pieces.
3. Cut tomatoes and onions and blanch with salt water (1 minute).
4. Cut the feta cheese into small cubes.
5. Mix zucchini with feta, tomatoes, onions, boiled eggs, add olives, and basil.

46. Golden Berry Smoothie with Banana and Turmeric

Ingredients
- 8 drops of TABASCO Green Jalapeño Sauce
- 50 ml of pineapple juice
- 50 ml of coconut water
- 25 ml of coconut milk
- A handful of spinach
- 6 coriander leaves
- 3 pineapple slices
- 5 ml of sugar syrup (depending on pineapple sweetness)

Preparation
Mix all ingredients in a blender and pour into a tall glass.

47. Roast Turkey with Spice Mix

Ingredients
- 1/4 cup yellow sugar
- 1/4 cup sweet paprika or paprika
- 2 tbsp dried oregano
- 2 tbsp dry thyme
- 1 tbsp chilli flakes (optional)

For turkey roast
- 1 turkey leg about 1.5kg
- 5 tbsp spice mix

Preparation
1. Mix all ingredients and place in a jar.
2. Place the turkey leg in a pyrex and season it with 5 tablespoons of the spice mixture. Cover the pyrex tightly with aluminium foil and bake at 180°C for about 1h30. At the end of this time, remove the foil and let the meat toast a little.
3. Serve the roast turkey with chips or rice and a green salad.
4. Use the spice mix to season pork or poultry for roasting and as a grill seasoning.

CHAPTER 9: Seafood recipes

48. Asparagus And Mixed Salad

Ingredients for 4 people
- Desalted cod 300 gr Metapontino
- strawberries 100 gr
- Asparagus 50 gr
- Arugula 20 gr
- Borage flowers 10 gr
- Yellow pepper 10 gr
- Fresh broad beans 20 gr
- Oil ex. Virgin of Ferrandina 100 gr
- Salt of maldon to taste lemon 4 slices

For the Dressing
- 1 Strawberries 100 gr
- Mint 10 gr Oil
- ex. virgin of Ferrandina 50 gr
- 2 Basil 50 gr
- Oil ex. Virgin of Ferrandina 50 gr.

Preparation
1. Desalinate the cod for at least 24 hours. Slice thinly with a knife and season with extra virgin olive oil. Clean and wash the strawberries with the rest of the vegetables, cut each vegetable into a different shape.
2. The strawberry must be cut into wedges, put everything in a bowl and mix gently, thus creating the salad that will accompany the cod.

For the dressing
3. Blend strawberries, oil, and mint in a special glass. Repeat the same preparation with the basil and the oil for the second dressing.
4. Arrange the slices of cod in a shallow dish, place the salad on top and season with both dressing, then add a few slices of lemon.

49. Cuttlefish Salad In Sweet And Sour Sauce

Ingredients for 2 people
- 550g of fresh cuttlefish
- 30g of raisins
- 20g of pine nuts
- 80g of oil
- 60g of vinegar rose grapes
- Salt to taste
- Parsley in leaves
- 1 head of radicchio

Preparation
1. Clean the cuttlefish and blanch in the water, the fins and the weave take longer. Cool and cut into julienne strips.
2. Clean the radicchio and cut it thinly.
3. In a steel bowl mix cuttlefish, radicchio, raisins, pine nuts, vinegar, oil, salt and a teaspoon of sugar.
4. Leave to marinate and flavor. Serve in a radicchio leaf. Decorate with parsley leaves.

50. Coronello Carpaccio And Dried Cherry Tomatoes

Ingredients
- Coronello (stockfish fillet) 500gr.
- Dried cherry tomatoes
- Black olives
- Extra virgin olive oil
- White pepper
- Capers "lacrimelle"
- Pomegranate or wild strawberries (depending on the season)

Preparation
1. The main component of this dish, but like all dishes, in addition to the freshness of any Ingredients, consists in the high quality of the

stockfish and in the right salting, otherwise you risk upsetting the simplicity of the dish itself.
2. The Coronello is peeled and the dish is mounted as if the gills were so many petals. It is a kind of tapenade of olives and cherry tomatoes and rests harmoniously on the coronello petals, together with the desalted capers.
3. Decorate the whole with pomegranate grains or with the pickled strawberries.

51. Flag Fish Roll With Smoked Provola

Ingredients for 4 people
- 2 kg of fish flag
- 150g smoked cheese
- bread grated
- extra-virgin olive oil
- salt, capers, garlic, and parsley
- Fillet the flag fish, making 30 cm fillets each.

Preparation
1. Compose the filling with a smoked provola nut, grated bread, capers, and minced garlic, wrap the fillets on themselves, bread them in the breadcrumbs. Bake at a temperature of 180° for about 5-7 minutes.
2. Pour a drizzle of extra virgin olive oil over the fillets and decorate with parsley leaves.

52. Spaghetti Marinara

Ingredients for 4 people
- Fresh or peeled San Marzano tomato 500 gr
- Black Gaeta olives 50 gr
- Desalinated capers 50 gr
- Extra virgin olive oil 80 gr
- Garlic 1 clove
- Oregano, salt to taste

- Spaghetti 350 gr

Preparation
1. Let the garlic go in the oil.
2. Remove it blond. Add the tomatoes, olives, capers and cook for a quarter of an hour.
3. Taste for salt.
4. Lower the pasta and remove it al dente. Add the spaghetti to the sauce and add plenty of oregano.
5. Jump on the plate.

53. Vermicelli With Cuttlefish Ink

Ingredients for 4 people
- 320 grams of linguine, vermicelli or spaghetti, even spaghettoni
- 3 very fresh squid ink pockets
- 250 gr. of cuttlefish
- 1 clove of garlic
- A very fresh lemon
- Extra virgin olive oil
- Fresh mint leaves

Preparation
1. Clean the cuttlefish well, peel them and carefully collect the black bags and set them aside. Brown in a large pan 8 tablespoons of extra virgin olive oil with the whole garlic and just crushed, pour the well-dried cuttlefish cut into small pieces and fry for 2 minutes.
2. At the same time cook the vermicelli or spaghetti or even spaghetti in abundant salted water.
3. In a bowl mix the cuttlefish black pasta in very little cooking water and pour it into the pan with the cuttlefish sauce, mixing well.
4. Strain the pasta al dente with a couple of minutes in advance and finish cooking by sautéing it in the pan with the dressing of the cuttlefish and the black, 2 drops of lemon each and, if necessary, add the pasta cooking water.

54. Ribbons With Thalli And Tuna

<u>Ingredients</u> for 2 people
- 200g of ribbons
- 200g of zucchini seeds
- 100g of tuna Callipo reserve gold
- 2 tablespoon of olive oil
- pepper
- garlic

<u>Preparation</u>
1. While the pasta is cooking, take the thalli clean and cut into strips, pass them quickly in boiling water.
2. On a frying pan make the garlic sweat and then remove it.
3. Add the thalli, Turn quickly.
4. Drain the pasta al dente and then add it to the thalli
5. Another minute turn off the heat, add the tuna and turn over Pepate
6. You can serve

55. Bluefin Tuna At The Two Sesame

<u>Ingredients</u> for 2 people
- 180gr of Sicilian red tuna
- 30 gr white and black sesame mix
- 25 grams of avocado
- 25gr of eggplant
- 15g candied ginger
- 20 gr soy sauce
- Salt and pepper and oil to taste

<u>Preparation</u>
1. Fillet and clean the red tuna, cut it into fillets and pass it in sesame. Blanch the fillets over high heat and cut into medallions. Separately cut the aubergines into strips, fry them and marinate them in soy.
2. Cut the red onions and cook in sweet and sour sauce, peel the avocado and blend it with a little oil and a dash of lemon

3. Place the tuna medallions on the plate and add the aubergines, the candied ginger, the avocado quenelles, the micro-salad and the chervil and season with the soy sauce.

56. Escarole And Cetara Anchovies Pie With Raisins And Pine Nuts

Ingredients for 8 people
- 2 heads of endive
- extra virgin olive oil
- 24 black olives from Gaeta
- 20 capers from Pantelleria desalinated
- 50 grams of stale bread
- 10 grams of pine nuts
- 20 grams of raisins
- 16 fillets of desalted anchovies
- 2 cloves of Italian garlic
- prezzzemolo qb
- 2 eggs.

Preparation
1. In a saucepan put the garlic to fry with extra virgin olive oil.
2. As soon as the garlic turns blond, add the endive that you have previously washed and coarsely chopped.
3. When the endive is withered add black olives and capers that you have carefully washed and desalted and proceed with quick cooking.
4. Let cool and place in a container.
5. Add the bread cut into cubes and the eggs that will serve to tie it all together.
6. Take some oil molds and fill them with the endive and bake at 160 degrees for 10 minutes.
7. Apart from having put the raisins to soak and toasted the pine nuts.
8. Put the baked pie in a shallow dish, garnish with raisins and toasted pine nuts, add the salted anchovies, preferably Cetara and a sprinkling of parsley.

57. Shrimp Pie

Ingredients
- 250g of flour
- 200g of unsalted cold butter
- 1 teaspoon salt
- 3 tbsp water
- 2 tbsp olive oil
- 2 cloves garlic, minced
- 400g peeled clean shrimp
- 1 tomato without skin and without chopped seed
- 2 tbsp coconut milk
- 1 minced finger pepper
- salt
- ¼ cup sour cream
- 2 tbsp chopped cilantro
- 1 gem

Preparation
1. Put the flour in a bowl and add the diced butter.
2. Knead with fingertips until crumbly.
3. Add salt and, gradually, water until it turns into dough. Cover with plastic and refrigerate for 1 hour.
4. Heat a frying pan, sprinkle with olive oil and brown the garlic and prawns.
5. Add the tomatoes, sauté for a couple of minutes, then add coconut milk and pepper and cook for another two minutes.
6. Season with salt, add the cream, turn off the heat and add the cilantro. Set aside to cool.
7. To open the dough in portions and to cover the pancakes, to stuff with the shrimp and to cover with a circle of dough.
8. Brush with the yolk and bake in the preheated oven at 180 degrees for about 30 minutes or until golden brown.

58. Creamy Shrimp Oven Rice

Ingredients
- 2 tbsp olive oil
- 600g clean little shrimp
- 1 clove minced garlic
- 1 chopped seedless tomato
- 2 tbsp tomato extract
- 1 cup canned sour cream
- salt
- Black pepper
- ¼ cup chopped parsley
- 5 cups cooked rice
- 2 gems
- 1 jar (200g) of curd
- ½ cup grated Parmesan + ½ cup sprinkling

Preparation
1. Heat a skillet, sprinkle with olive oil, and brown the shrimp. Add the garlic, the chopped tomatoes, sauté for 2 minutes and add the tomato extract and then the cream, season with salt and pepper, turn off the heat and set aside.
2. In a bowl, combine rice, egg yolks, curd, and ½ cup Parmesan.
3. Cover the bottom of a previously oiled refractory with rice. Arrange the prawns, cover with parsley, and ½ cup Parmesan cheese.
4. Bake in the preheated oven at 180 degrees for about 25 minutes or until browned the cheese.

59. Shrimp in the pumpkin

Ingredients
- 1 large pumpkin
- 8 cloves garlic, minced
- 1 ½ minced onion
- Black pepper to taste
- Salt to taste

- 3 tablespoons olive oil + braised olive oil
- 1kg clean, fresh shrimp
- 2 chopped tomatoes
- ½ cup of passata
- ¼ bunch of coriander
- 2 seedless minced finger peppers
- 1 can of sour cream
- 1 cup of curd
- 100g grated mozzarella cheese

Preparation
1. Open the pumpkin, remove the seeds. Reserve.
2. Knead 5 cloves of garlic with ½ onion, black pepper, salt, and olive oil.
3. Rub this paste inside the pumpkin, cover and bake at 180 degrees for 30 minutes.
4. Season the shrimps with salt, black pepper, and lemon juice.
5. In a hot skillet with a drizzle of olive oil, brown the prawns, season with salt and pepper, and set aside.
6. Sauté the remaining onion, garlic and add the tomatoes and cook for 10 minutes.
7. Add the coriander, the pepper, the cream, the curd, the prawns, and correct the salt.
8. Arrange the shrimp with the sauce inside the pumpkin and mix it with the cooked pumpkin from the inside.
9. Top with grated mozzarella cheese.
10. Bake in the preheated oven for 20 minutes or until browned.

60. Seafood Noodles

Ingredients
- Braised olive oil
- 4 cloves garlic, minced
- 300g of clean squid cut into rings
- 200g mussel without shell
- 200g shellless volley
- 10 clean prawns

- 150g of dried tomatoes
- salt to taste
- black pepper to taste
- 500g of pre-cooked noodles
- ½ pack of watercress
- ½ Lemon Juice
- parsley to taste

Preparation
1. In olive oil, sauté the garlic and add the squid, the mussel, the shrimp, and the shrimp.
2. Add the dried tomatoes and season with salt and pepper.
3. Add the noodles, watercress, season with lemon juice, and parsley.

61. Potato Dumpling with Shrimp

Ingredients
- 500g of pink potatoes
- 1 egg
- salt to taste
- 1 tbsp chopped parsley
- 2 tablespoons flour + flour for handling and breading
- 10 units of clean giant tailed shrimp
- black pepper to taste
- ½ packet of chopped cilantro
- 3 tablespoons palm oil
- 4 lemon juice
- frying oil

Preparation
1. Put the potato to cook for 40 minutes.
2. When very tender, remove from heat, let cool and mash potatoes already peeled.
3. Add the egg and mix well, season with salt and parsley and add the flour. Set aside in the fridge for 2 hours.
4. Make small transverse cuts on the belly of the shrimp, without cutting to the end. Season the shrimp with salt, black pepper,

chopped coriander, palm oil, and lemon juice. Leave marinating for 15 minutes.
5. Take a portion of the potato flour dough in your hands and shape around a shrimp leaving the tail out.
6. Rinse flour again and fry in hot oil until golden.

62. Creamy Shrimp Cone

Ingredients
- Braised olive oil
- 3 cloves minced garlic
- 400g Shrimp Sauce (clean and peeled)
- 2 tablespoons tomato paste
- 1 cup of coconut milk
- Salt to taste
- 1 minced finger pepper
- 2 tbsp chopped cilantro
- 100g grated mozzarella cheese
- 100g of bread bran

Preparation
1. In olive oil, sauté the garlic until it gives off an aroma.
2. Add the shrimp.
3. Add tomato extract, coconut milk, and reduce for 10 minutes over medium heat.
4. Season with salt, pepper, ginger, and chopped coriander.
5. Arrange in peels or ramekins, arrange portions of mozzarella cheese and portions of breadcrumbs and bake 180 degrees for 20 minutes or until browned.

63. Shrimp cocktail

Ingredients
- 10 clean, peeled and tailed GG prawns
- salt
- Black pepper
- 150g chopped clean medium shrimp

- 100ml of cold milk
- 1 cup olive oil
- ½ clove garlic
- 1 cup ketchup
- ½ cup of pepper jelly
- 1 tbsp brandy
- 2 tbsp English sauce
- 1 tbsp chopped cilantro + 1 tbsp to garnish

Preparation
1. To heat a frying pan, to arrange GG prawns, to the season with salt and pepper and to broil until golden, to reserve.
2. In the same skillet, quickly sauté the chopped shrimps, season with salt and pepper, and set aside.
3. In a blender, beat the chilled milk and gradually turn the olive oil until it is consistent.
4. Add the garlic clove, salt, and ketchup.
5. To arrange in a bowl and to add the pepper jelly, the brandy, the English sauce, the coriander, and the minced prawns. Mix and bring it to the fridge.
6. When cold, serve the sauce in bowls with the prawns, sprinkle cilantro and serve.

64. Shrimp Basket

Ingredients
- 200g of filo pastry
- 1 tablespoon melted butter
- 400g medium shrimp
- 2 tbsp olive oil
- salt
- Black pepper
- 450g of cream cheese
- 100g of sour cream
- 2 tbsp lemon juice
- 1 tsp lemon zest

Preparation
1. Cut squares of filo pastry, place two squares of dough in each muffin pan, brush with butter and bake in a preheated oven at 180 degrees for about 20 minutes or until golden brown.
2. Heat a frying pan, sprinkle with oil, add portions of shrimps, season with salt and pepper and brown for approximately 3 minutes. Repeat the process with all the shrimp and set aside.
3. Mix cream cheese with sour cream, add lemon juice, pepper, and prawns ¾.
4. Arrange portions of cream in filo baskets and garnish with remaining shrimp and lemon zest.

65. Shrimp Stash

Ingredients
- Braised olive oil
- 400g of shrimp
- 1 chopped onion
- 1 clove minced garlic
- 1 minced pepper
- 2 tbsp tomato extract
- Salt to taste
- 200g of curd
- 2 tbsp chopped parsley
- 250g of baroa potatoes
- 100g of sour cream
- 150g grated mozzarella cheese

Preparation
1. Over high heat, sauté the shrimp slightly and add and onion, the minced garlic, and the finger pepper.
2. Add the tomato paste, a pinch of salt, then the curd, and the chopped parsley. Reserve.
3. To cook the baron potatoes in boiling water.
4. To mash the baron potatoes and to add the cream. Season with salt. If necessary, use a mixer to make the puree smooth. Reserve.

5. Arrange the shrimp in a refractory form, arrange the mozzarella cheese and cover with the manioc puree on top.
6. Bake at 200 degrees for 15 minutes

CHAPTER 10: Poultry Recipe

66. Chicken Pops

<u>Ingredients</u> for 2 people
- 1 kilo of chicken (tenderloins)
- 2 eggs
- 300 grams of breadcrumbs or panko
- Black pepper
- Oil
- Salt

<u>Preparation</u>
1. Cut the chicken tenderloins into small squares and salt them.
2. In a bowl, beat the eggs. In another bowl, we put the 300 grams of panko. Meanwhile, heat extra virgin olive oil in a pan or fryer.
3. Batter the chicken squares in egg and then passes them through the panko. When the oil is very hot, you should fry.
4. Let the chicken pops drain on a plate with paper towels. Subsequently, present and accompany with some sauce to taste.

67. Roasted Chicken In Cocotte

<u>Ingredients</u> for 1 chicken
- 1 chicken of 2 kilos
- 2 carrots
- 2 large tomatoes
- 1 large onion
- 30 milliliters of fruity white wine
- 70 milliliters of bird broth
- Fresh parsley
- Extra virgin olive oil
- White wine vinegar
- Pepper
- Salt

Preparation
1. Preheat the oven to about 200 degrees Celsius.
2. Clean the chicken of any remaining fat and feathers.
3. Peel the carrots, tomatoes and scallions.
4. Cut tomatoes and scallions into large pieces and sliced carrots. Place the cut vegetables inside the cocotte or cast iron casserole.
5. Season to taste and pour a dash of extra virgin olive oil and a few drops of vinegar on the vegetable.
6. Season the chicken, both inside and out, and place inside the casserole with the breast part on the vegetables.
7. Clean and crush the garlic in a mortar together with two sprigs of fresh parsley. We add 4 tablespoons of extra virgin olive oil and three of vinegar.
8. Mix the wine and the bird broth. Stir and water the chicken with this combination.
9. Introduce the cocotte or casserole with all the ingredients inside the oven at medium height. Let bake with the cocotte covered for 45 minutes at 200 degrees Celsius.
10. Turn the chicken over after 45 minutes, cover the cocotte and put it back in the oven for 50 minutes at 180 degrees.
11. Prick and insert a long needle or fine utensil into different parts of the chicken to check if the chicken is already cooked.
12. Uncover the pot if we have verified that the chicken is already roasted, at this time change the function of the oven to grill mode and raise the temperature to about 220 degrees.
13. Let the skin brown and crisp for a few minutes. Observe that the skin acquires a tan tone, and then it will be.
14. Remove the chicken from the oven, carve and serve while it is hot.

68. Chilindron Chicken

Ingredients
- 1 chopped chicken
- 4 ripe tomatoes
- 1 large red pepper
- 1 large green pepper
- 4 garlic cloves

- 1 large onion
- 100 grams of serrano ham
- 250 milliliters of white wine
- Extra virgin olive oil
- Salt

Preparation

1. Heat a large stream of olive oil in the pan, peel two cloves of garlic and cook until golden brown. When they have taken the color, remove them from the pan since what is sought is that the flavor remains in it.
2. Remove the skin from the chicken and wash it well. Already chopped, put it to cook in the same pan where you have browned the garlic and add a little salt.
3. Fry it at medium temperature and be patient until it turns golden. Once ready, remove it from the pan and reserve.
4. In a large pot, heat a generous stream of extra virgin olive oil. Chop the garlic, cut the large onion into julienne and add them to the saucepan so that they are poached over medium heat.
5. When the onion begins to brown, wash the peppers, cut them into strips and add them to the pot so that everything is poached together.
6. You should be aware and stir so that the ingredients do not stick to the bottom of the pot you should be aware and stir so that the ingredients do not stick to the bottom of the pot
7. Wash the tomatoes, peel them and cut them in tacos. Also, chop the ham and when the peppers are al dente add only the ham to the pot.
8. After a couple of minutes, add the tomato pieces. Cook all ingredients over medium-low heat for 8 minutes. You should be pending and remove so that they are not stuck to the bottom of the pot.
9. After the indicated time, add the chopped chicken to the pot and pour over 250 milliliters of white wine. Stir everything well so that the sauce is distributed by the chicken and let it cook all over medium-low heat for another 8 minutes.
10. If you are a sauce lover and you want to have plenty, add a little more water so that the stew is not very dry. You can also add some

thyme or rosemary that will give the chicken another special touch.
11. When the 8 minutes have passed and your chicken is ready, rectify and add more salt if you consider it necessary.
12. Remove the pot from the heat and your stew will be ready to sit. Serve it immediately after removing it from the heat so that it is hot and freshly made.

69. Moroccan Roast Turkey

Ingredients

- 1 turkey (leg)
- 1 tablespoon cumin (rash hanout)
- 1 glass of virgin olive oil
- 1 glass of white wine
- 1 tablespoon salt
- 1 tablespoon of pepper
- 1 large garlic
- 1 glass of parsley
- 1 glass of peppermint
- 3 medium potatoes

Preparations
1. The first thing to do is to clean the leg correctly. This corresponds to the chicken's thigh and we have taken this piece and not the breast since it is much more tasty and juicy. If we do it with the breast, we run the risk of being dry.
2. We have to be careful when cleaning the leg. First, we have to separate the cartilage and also clean thoroughly by rubbing with water there will be no pen left. When we have it ready, we will make some superficial cuts so that when it comes to spreading the ingredients the meat takes on the flavor.
3. We put the rasp of hanout, virgin olive oil, white wine, salt, pepper, garlic, and peppermint in the blender and make a homogeneous mixture.
4. If we do not have a mixer we can do it with some rods or even with a fork, it does not matter. With that emulsion, we will spread

the turkey's leg on both sides making the mixture enter the surface cuts.
5. While we put the oven to heat. The next step is the garnish; here we have chosen potatoes as it is a perfect combination with poultry.
6. What you have to do is peel them and then cut them into slices a centimeter thick. We are also going to impregnate these potatoes with the mixture of ingredients with which we have coated the turkey.
7. Finally, we will take a baking dish. If you wish at the bottom you can put some butter spread with your hands and then put the potatoes.
8. On top, we will place the leg and if we have enough we will put the mixture that we have made of ingredients. With the hot oven, we put the source and we will have it at 180 degrees about two hours approximately.
9. From time to time we can open the oven and serve over the leg the juice that is released at the bottom of the fountain.
10. In addition, if we see the leg on the outside quite tanned, we can put a silver paper on top so that the inside part is done well.
11. So it only remains to place and taste this delicious roast of Moroccan turkey.

70. Chicken With Mushrooms Cream

Ingredients
- 2 large chicken breasts
- 200 grams of rolled mushrooms
- 1 small onion
- 125 milliliters of white wine
- 125 milligrams of chicken broth
- 4 tablespoons of cream for cooking
- Oil
- Salt
- Pepper

Preparation

1. We prepare the breasts to taste. Being large we can cut them in half and leave them whole to make 4 dishes or we can cut them into slices from the beginning so that the preparation of the recipe is much faster.
2. We will season them to taste and reserve until we begin to cook them.
3. We will chop as small as possible with a knife a small onion. We will use a pan large enough to fit all the ingredients when we mix them.
4. We will heat it with a drizzle of oil and begin to poach the onion for a few minutes until it is transparent and somewhat golden brown. We will reserve.
5. In that same pan, rectifying with the oil if necessary, we will skip the chicken pieces so that they begin to be made for a few minutes.
6. It does not matter if it is still raw because we will reserve next to the onion and in the pan, we will start making the mushrooms. We will add a little more oil until they are made and browned.
7. With the mushrooms, the onion, and the chicken half-done we will proceed to make the cream that will give this preparation all the flavour.
8. We will first add the white wine, letting it cook with the mushrooms so that the alcohol evaporates.
9. We let it cook for a couple of minutes we will add the chicken broth and, after stirring a little, we will continue cooking so that the broth is gradually reduced.
10. Add the onion and chicken to the pan and let it finish with the broth. We will add the tablespoons of cream to cook and stir well so that the sauce that we have made from the broth and the wine becomes much creamier.
11. You can also add some aromatic herb such as rosemary to give it a touch of different flavor
12. We will let cook for 5 to 10 minutes until we see that the sauce has been reduced and that the chicken is completely done. We can take as a single dish or also with a little salad or mash to accompany.

Note
If you do not want this recipe to remain creamy, discard the cream and so you can enjoy a much lighter sauce.

71. Garlic Chicken

<u>Ingredients</u> for 4 people
- 1 chicken cut
- 7 garlic cloves
- 2 bay leaves
- 200 milliliters of white wine from Jerez
- Olive oil
- Salt
- Pepper

<u>Preparation</u>
1. We will buy the chicken already sliced from the butcher shop or, in the case of knowing how to chop it, we can also do it at home.
2. We will try to remove the fat from the meat so that the result is not too greasy. Chicken skin also brings more fat to this dish but if you like to take it, you can leave it.
3. Once the chicken is ready, we will prepare the casserole where we will cook all the ingredients. We will add oil until we cover completely; the base of the casserole and it is just a little thick.
4. We will select 7 cloves of garlic and, without peeling, we will sauté in the pan over medium heat so that the garlic begins to become soft trying not to burn. You can also chop them to cook them more crumbled.
5. That way, the oil will be flavored thanks to the garlic and leave that taste in the chicken. We will reserve the garlic outside the fire and add the chicken pieces next to the bay leaves.
6. We can add other aromatic herbs to taste such as rosemary or thyme. We will cook for approximately 15 minutes, letting the chicken become completely tender and crispy on the outside.
7. The garlic in this recipe can be left whole or chop it to taste
8. After that time, we will add the garlic cloves and the white wine, allowing the time necessary for the alcohol to evaporate and the wine to reduce as much as possible until it leaves a more or less thick sauce.
9. We can prepare a salad to place in the center and thus accompany this delicious chicken dish that we will serve very hot.

Note
You can add a little chicken broth to the sauce, letting it reduce with the wine.

72. Lemon Chicken

Ingredients for 4 people
- 2 chicken breasts (whole)
- 2 eggs
- 50 grams of cornstarch
- Breadcrumbs
- 4 lemons
- 1 tablespoon of sugar

Preparation
1. The first thing we will do is prepare the breasts. They will not be filleted so we can cut them into small, bite-sized pieces so we can enjoy them better.
2. But the treatment we give to the breast has to be to taste. If you prefer to fillet and serve it whole, you can also.
3. We will put the cornstarch, tahe breadcrumbs, and the two beaten eggs in three different containers in order to breach them, just as we would do to make croquettes or other similar elaboration.
4. We will pass the pieces of the breast through the cornstarch, followed by the egg and finally the breadcrumbs. Once we have the breaded pieces, we fry them in abundant hot oil in a pan for a few minutes back and forth.
5. We will reserve on absorbent paper to get rid of the remaining oil.
6. For the sauce, we will squeeze the juice of 4 lemons making sure that no bones fall. We will reserve if we want, some small slices of lemon to decorate.
7. In a small saucepan over medium heat, we will add the lemon juice with the spoonful of sugar, moving with a wooden spoon to dilute it.
8. In a glass with water, add a spoonful of cornstarch and stir until dissolved. We will add it to the saucepan and boil until we have the desired consistency.

9. At the time of serving, we will place the pieces of breaded chicken and we will throw the sauce on top or we will place it in a small container to wet the pieces to the pleasure. Do you dare with this simple recipe?

Note
We can make the grilled breasts if we do not want this dish to have many calories.

73. Chicken curry

Ingredients for 4 people
- 4 chicken breasts
- 4 garlic
- 1 pinch ginger
- 1 clove of garlic
- 1 onion (medium)
- 50 grams of almonds
- 1 tablespoon tomato (fried or crushed)
- 250 milliliters of coconut milk
- 2 tablespoons curry
- 1 teaspoon cumin
- 1 teaspoon cumin
- Salt
- Pepper

Preparation
1. In a frying pan with a little background, we poach the garlic, onion, garlic, almonds, and ginger well chopped.
2. After about 10 minutes, add the tomato and spices. Remove and sauté so that this sauce is cooked well.
3. Season the sliced breasts with a little more curry and season to taste before adding them to the pan.
4. Sauté for a few minutes before adding coconut milk. Let simmer to reduce.
5. We serve.

74. Chicken wings with tomato sauce and mince

Ingredients
- 1 kg of chicken wings
- 800g canned tomatoes
- 1 tbsp red pepper
- 1 tsp black pepper
- salt to taste
- 2 tbsp lemon juice
- 1 tbsp honey
- 1 tsp chromite
- 1 tbsp oil
- 400g minced mixture (60 / 40)
- 150 ml chicken broth

Preparation
1. Mix the preserved peeled tomato cubes with red and black pepper, salt, lemon juice, and honey. Put the wings in this marina to soak for a few hours.
2. Remove them, drain them and grill them on both sides until golden and the meat is completely cooked.
3. During this time, prepare the sauce. Cut the bromide into cubes and fry it in the oil until soft. Add the mince and fry until ready.
4. Pour broth and bring to a boil. Add the marinade and cook for a few minutes. Serve chicken wings warm, drizzle with tomato sauce with mince. Sprinkle them with fresh parsley if desired.

75. Chicken medallions

Ingredients
- 500g chicken fillet
- 50 grams of cheese
- 1/2 tsp. + 2 tsp flour
- 200 ml of tomato juice
- 100g canned mushrooms

- 150 grams of ham
- 1 pc egg
- 2 pc slice of bread
- pepper
- salt

Preparation
1. Fill the chicken fillet lightly with a piece of yellow cheese on each steak.
2. Then roll into a ball and roll into flour (1/2 hour).
3. Fry on both sides until red.
4. The slices are dipped in the broken egg and fried.
5. Prepare the sauce by frying the mushrooms, ham, flour, and tomato juice (if you find it very thick, add some water).
6. Season with salt and pepper and simmer for a few minutes.
7. In a serving platter, place the fried fillet, fillet on it, and pour over the tomato sauce.

76. Chicken fillet

Ingredients
- 1 kg chicken fillet
- 200g flour
- 200g bread crumbs
- 5 eggs
- 60g universal seasoning

For sauce
- 1 packet of mayonnaise
- 1/2 cup yoghurt
- 2-3 cloves garlic
- 2-3 twigs basil
- pinch salt

Preparation
1. Cut chicken strips lengthwise.

2. Sprinkle with a universal spice, roll in flour, egg, breadcrumbs, and each strip is formed between the palms of the hands like a cigar.
3. Fry in heated oil until golden.
4. The sauce is cooked, and the garlic, basil, and some of the milk are mixed with a blender.
5. Mayonnaise, salt, and other milk are added.
6. Stir until a homogeneous mixture.
7. Pour over the sauce and serve with a slice of lemon.

77. Chicken rolls with cheese

Ingredients
- 1 kg chicken fillet
- 1 carrot
- 200g cheese
- garlic to taste
- 2-3 tbsp oil
- salt to taste
- ground black pepper to taste
- 3 tbsp mayonnaise

Preparation
1. Cut each chicken fillet lengthwise, beat it with a meat hammer to make it thinner, and rub it with salt and pepper. Allow standing for 20 minutes.
2. Grind the carrots and the cheese and mix them with crushed garlic and a tablespoon of mayonnaise.
3. Put the cheese filling on each fillet, roll, and tighten.
4. Fry the rolls in the heated oil until red, remove them, remove the thread and arrange them in a pan.
5. Pour them in half with water and grease them with the remaining mayonnaise. Bake the rolls in a moderate oven for about 20 minutes.

78. Chicken timbal with cottage cheese and spinach

Ingredients
- 200g Olympus curd
- 50g breadcrumbs 2 pcs. chicken breast fillets of very thin fillets
- 300g spinach
- 100g grated cheese Olympus Olympus
- oil for spreading
- salt, pepper

For sauce
- 200g Olympus milk
- 100g roasted red pepper
- dill, mint, salt, pepper

Preparation
1. For timbals, grease the shapes (for caramel or Brulee). Sprinkle the bottom and walls with breadcrumbs.
2. Place the salmon, and black pepper flavoured so that they cover the bottom and walls of each shape. The fillets should be longer in order for them to be slammed over the filling and to get tumbles.
3. Stew the spinach in a little butter and olive oil. Season with salt and pepper. Pull the pan off the stove and add the curd and cheese. Stir well.
4. Pour the spinach mixture into each tray. Move the chicken fillets to close the tambourine. Sprinkle with breadcrumbs and bake at 160-180 degrees in a preheated oven for 40 minutes or until ready.
5. To prepare the pepper cream, paste all the products and season.

79. Chicken with rice in the oven

Ingredients
- 3L of water
- 700g chicken legs (upper and lower)
- 1 tbsp salt

- 3 tbsp butter or oil
- 1 bromide onion
- 2 carrots
- 1 red pepper
- 200g (1 h) rice
- salt
- ground black pepper
- savoury
- parsley

Preparation
1. For the recipe "Chicken with Oven Rice" in a large saucepan boil the water together with 1 tablespoon salt.
2. Start chicken legs and cook for about 30-35 minutes.
3. The chicken legs are removed and deboned, and the broth is cooked and strained.
4. In a large frying pan, the oil burns.
5. Add the peeled and sliced onions and carrots.
6. Simmer until soft for about 5 minutes and add chopped pepper.
7. Cook for another 5 minutes, then pour the rice.
8. Fry until whitening.
9. Meat and rice are distributed in a refractory pan.
10. Sprinkled with savoury, salt, and ground black pepper.
11. Pour over 3 hours of strained broth.
12. The oven is heated to 220° C.
13. Chicken with rice in the oven is baked for 25-30 minutes or until the rice has absorbed all the water and is left with only fat.
14. The dish "Chicken with Oven Rice" is distributed on plates and served, sprinkled, if desired, with finely chopped parsley.

CHAPTER 11: DESSERT RECIPES

80. Toasted Almond Ambrosia

This southern classic provides 45 milligrams of vitamin C, equivalent to more than 75 percent of the recommended daily intake.

Ingredients
- 1/2 cup sliced almonds
- 1/2 cup unsweetened grated coconut
- 1 small pineapple, diced (approximately 3 cups)
- 5 oranges, in segments
- 2 red apples, heartless and diced
- 1 peeled banana, cut lengthwise in half and sliced transversely
- 2 tablespoons Sherry Cream wine
- Fresh mint leaves to decorate

Preparation
1. Heat the oven to 325 ° F (160 ° C). Place the almonds on a baking sheet and bake; Stir a few times until golden brown and give off its aroma, for about 10 minutes.
2. Transfer immediately to a plate to cool. Add the coconut to the tray and bake, stirring frequently, until lightly browned, for about 10 minutes.
3. Transfer immediately to a plate to cool.
4. In a large bowl, mix the pineapple, oranges, apples, banana, and sherry. Stir gently to mix well.
5. Place the fruit mixture evenly in different individual bowls. Sprinkle evenly with roasted almonds and coconut, and garnish with mint. Serve immediately.

Nutritional Information - Composition Amount (g) CDR (%) for 8 servings
Calories: 177
Total Fat: 5 g

Saturated Fat: 1 g
Trans fa:t Minimum amount
Monounsaturated Fat: 2 g
Cholesterol: 0mg
Sodium: 2mg
Total carbohydrate: 30 g
Dietary fiber: 6 g
Total sugars: 21 g
Added sugars: 0 g
Protein: 3 g

81. Apricot Biscotti

This cookie with double cooking is a classic to accompany coffee or tea. Whole wheat and walnuts provide the mineral manganese and the antioxidant selenium.

Ingredients
- 3/4 cup bran flour (whole wheat)
- 3/4 cup common flour (white)
- 1/4 cup brown sugar, very compact
- 1 teaspoon baking powder
- 2 eggs, lightly beaten
- 2 tablespoons 1 percent low-fat milk
- 2 tablespoons canola oil
- 2 tablespoons dark honey
- 1/2 teaspoon almond extract
- 2/3 cup chopped dried apricots
- 1/4 cup large chopped almonds

Preparation
1. Heat the oven to 350 ° F (175 ° C).
2. In a large bowl, place the flour, brown sugar and baking powder.
3. Beat until mixed. Add eggs, milk, canola oil, honey, and almond extract.
4. Stir with a wooden spoon until the dough begins to integrate. Add almonds and chopped apricots. With floured hands, mix the dough until the ingredients are well integrated.

5. Place the dough on a large sheet of plastic wrap and form a crushed roll 12 inches (30 cm) long, 3 inches (7.5 cm) wide and about 1 inch (2.5 cm) by hand.
6. High Lift the plastic wrap and invert the dough in a non-stick baking sheet. Bake for 25-30 minutes, until lightly browned.
7. Transfer it to another baking sheet and let it cool for 10 minutes. Leave the oven at 350 ° F (175 ° C).
8. Place the cold dough on a cutting board. With a serrated knife, cut transversely into 24 1/2 inch (1 cm) wide portions. Place the portions with the cut down on the baking sheet.
9. Bake again for 15-20 minutes, until crispy. Go to a rack and let cool completely.
10. Store in an airtight container.

Nutritional Information - Composition Amount (g) CDR (%) for 1 cookie
Calories: 75
Total Fat: 2 g
Saturated Fat: Minimum Quantity
Monounsaturated Fat: 1 g
Cholesterol: 15mg
Sodium:17mg
Total carbohydrate: 12 g
Dietary fiber: 1 g
Total sugars: 6 g
Added sugars: 2 g
Protein: 2 g

82. Apple And Berry Cobbler

This recipe is a lighter, fresher version of the traditional fruit cake.

Ingredients
- 1 cup fresh raspberries
- 1 cup fresh blueberries
- 2 cups chopped apples
- 2 tablespoons turbinado sugar or brown sugar

- 1/2 teaspoon ground cinnamon
- 1 teaspoon lemon zest
- 2 teaspoons lemon juice
- 1 1/2 tablespoon cornstarch
- For the coating:
- 1 large egg white
- 1/4 cup soy milk
- 1/4 teaspoon salt
- 1/2 teaspoon of vanilla
- 1 1/2 tablespoon of turbinado sugar or brown sugar
- 3/4 cup pastry wholemeal flour

Preparation
1. Preheat the oven to 350 ° F (175 ° C). Lightly cover 6 individual baking pans with oil spray.
2. In a medium bowl, add the raspberries, blueberries, apples, sugar, cinnamon, lemon zest, and lemon juice. Stir to mix well. Add the cornstarch and stir until dissolved.
3. In a separate bowl, add the egg white and beat until lightly beaten. Add soy milk, salt, vanilla, sugar, and baking flour. Stir to mix well.
4. Divide the berry mixture evenly between the prepared dishes. Pour the mixture over each dish. Organize the casseroles in a large baking dish and place in the oven.
5. Bake the berries until they are tender and the topping is golden brown, about 30 minutes. Serve warm.

Nutritional Information - Composition Amount (g) CDR (%) for 6 servings
Calories: 136
Total Fat: Minimum amount
Saturated Fat: Minimum Quantity
Trans Fat: 0 g
Monounsaturated Fat: Minimum amount
Cholesterol: 0mg
Sodium: 111mg
Total carbohydrate: 31 g
Dietary fiber: 4 g

Added sugars: 7 g
Protein: 3 g

83. Chocolate Mascarpone

<u>Ingredients</u> for 4 cups or for putting 1 cake
- 250ml. fondant cream (well chilled)
- 250g. Mascarpone cheese
- 200 g. Dark chocolate
- 4 tablespoons powdered sugar

<u>Preparation</u>
1. Applying cream, we dissolve chocolate in a water bath - i.e. place the chocolate in a glass bowl.
2. Place the bowl on a pot with boiling water - so that the bottom of the bowl does not touch the water.
3. Leave the melted chocolate to cool (until it is not hot, only slightly warm).
4. Whip cream.
5. Mix mascarpone cheese with a mixer with powdered sugar.
6. Without stopping the mixer - we add chocolate to the cheese (gently pour in a small stream).
7. Mix until smooth.
8. Add whipped cream to the chocolate mass.
9. Then mix - manually or with a mixer at low speed until we get a uniform, creamy, thick consistency.
10. To get a nice-looking dessert - apply the cream to the cup using the sleeve to decorate the cakes.
11. We store the ready cream in the fridge.

84. Almond Ricotta Spread

Preparation Time: 30 minutes

<u>Ingredients</u>
- 200 gr. raw and unsalted almonds
- 100 gr. raw and unsalted cashews

- 2 tablespoons lemon juice
- Sea salt at ease
- 1 tablespoon of yeast in "Titan" flakes (if you don't have a very fine grating, a little bit of "Violife" cheddar type cheese)
- Black pepper to taste
- Fresh herbs to taste (rosemary, parsley, dill, sage, thyme, coriander)

Preparation
1. Soak the nuts for a minimum of 8 hours overnight.
2. The next day, strain the nuts and process them with lemon juice, salt, flaked yeast (or very fine grated "Viollife" cheese) and pepper until a thick cream is formed.
3. Turn the processor on and off if necessary, and stir well so that everything is well integrated.
4. Some water can be added, but not in excess to prevent the dip from becoming too liquid. It should have the consistency of the traditional "pillory."
5. Rectify the salt and pepper again and add fresh herbs on top.

Note
This is a basic recipe that will serve you to use in various formats. For example, to fill ravioli, prepare cakes, use as a dip, spread sandwiches or simply spoon.

85. Baklava With Lemon Honey Syrup

Ingredients
- 400g of filo pastry
- 300g of walnuts
- 250g of pistachios
- 200g of butter
- 200g of sugar
- a tablespoon of lemon juice
- 2 tablespoons of honey
- 300 ml of water

Preparation

1. Melt the butter in a saucepan and let it cool, while chopping the pistachios and almonds together with two tablespoons of sugar.
2. Butter the pan, then spread the first sheet of phyllo dough, brush it with the melted butter and place a second and a third on it, still buttering.
3. After the third layer, place chopped walnuts and pistachios and start the process again: for every 3 sheets of buttered pasta, insert a layer of walnuts and pistachios until you finish with the filo pastry.
4. Bake at 180 ° for 15 minutes. Meanwhile, prepare the syrup, bring to a boil (over medium heat and stir constantly) the sugar, water, lemon juice, and honey.
5. Once cooked sprinkle the syrup baklava, let it cool and serve cut into diamonds and covered with chopped walnuts and pistachios.

86. Kourabiedes Greek Butter Cookies

Ingredients
- 150g raw almonds
- 155g soft butter (at room temperature)
- 70g caster sugar
- 2 egg yolks
- 300g flour 00
- 1/2 teaspoon baking powder
- Icing sugar to taste
- 20 whole cloves

Preparation
1. Bring a saucepan to boil with water.
2. When the water boils, add the almonds, cook for 10 minutes and then drain on a sheet of absorbent paper. Remove the almond skin.
3. Light the oven at 200 ° C, cover a baking sheet with baking paper and toast the almonds.
4. When they are well toasted, let them cool. Once cold, whisk it with a chopper. Do not reduce them to flour, but get a fine grain.
5. Whip the butter with the sugar, helping yourself with the electric whisk until you get froth.

6. Add the egg yolks and mix with the whisk until all the ingredients are mixed. Sift the flour and baking powder.
7. Add the flour, baking powder and chopped almonds to the dough.
8. Start kneading in the bowl, then move to a table and knead: it takes a little patience before the dough becomes compact.
9. As soon as you get compact dough, wrap it in plastic wrap and let it rest in the fridge for an hour.
10. As soon as this time has elapsed, preheat the oven to 180 ° C and cover a baking sheet with baking paper.
11. Make balls about the size of a walnut and place them on the baking tray, placing them at a distance of two cm from each other.
12. Press the center of each ball with the fingertips, so as to obtain a small furrow and bake for 20 minutes or until golden brown.
13. When baked, put a clove in the center of each cookie.
14. Let them cool and then sprinkle with plenty of icing sugar.

87. Fresh Cranberry Pie

<u>Ingredients</u>
- 1 ½ cup crumbled Graham crackers
- ¼ cup salt-free chopped pecans
- 1 ¾ cup Splenda Sweetener
- ½ cup non-hydrogenated salt-free margarine
- 1 ½ cup freshly picked cranberries
- 2 egg whites
- 1 tbsp. thawed apple juice concentrate
- 1 tbsp. vanilla extract
- 1 litre Cool Whip Whipped Topping, thawed

Cranberry Frosting
- ¼ cup Splenda Sweetener
- ¼ cup caster sugar
- 1 Tbsp. cornstarch
- ¾ cup fresh cranberries
- ¾ cup of water

<u>Preparation</u>

1. Preheat oven to 375 ° F (190 ° C).
2. Mix crumbled crackers, pecans, and ¾ cup of Splenda. Add the margarine, mix well, and arrange on a hinged mould pressing on the bottom and the sides. Bake dough for 6 minutes or until slightly browned let cool.
3. Mix the cranberries with 1 cup of Splenda. Let stand for 5 minutes. Add the egg whites, apple juice, and vanilla. Beat at low speed until foamy, and then beat at high speed for 5 to 8 minutes until mixture is firm.
4. Stir in the whipped topping in the cranberry mixture. Pour the mixture over the pre-cooked dough. Refrigerate at least 4 hours until the mixture is firm.
5. To make the icing, mix the sugar, Splenda, and cornstarch in a saucepan. Stir in cranberries and water. Cook, stirring until bubbles appear. Continue cooking, occasionally stirring until cranberry skin comes off. Use the mixture at room temperature. Do not refrigerate: the sauce may crystallize and become opaque.
6. Remove the tart from the pan and arrange on a serving platter, using a spoon, coat with icing.

88. Cocoa muffins with coffee

Ingredients
- 1/2 hour soft butter
- 1 egg
- 1 teaspoon sugar
- 1 teaspoon vanilla
- 1 -1/2 teaspoon flour
- 1 teaspoon baking soda
- salt
- 1/2 teaspoon cocoa
- 1/2 teaspoon yoghurt
- 1/3 teaspoon strong coffee

Preparation
1. Beat the butter with the sugar, add the egg and vanilla.
2. 2. Mix flour, baking soda, salt, cocoa separately.

3. 3. Add the dry ingredients of the parts together with the yoghurt and the coffee parts to the egg mixture.
4. Preheat the oven to 180 degrees, fill the muffin cups with 2/3 of the mixture and bake for 20-25 minutes. or until ready.
5. 3. For the glaze, I experimented and made it with liquid pastry cream / about 3/4 cup of tea / and a packet of 1 kg powdered sugar (I didn't get the whole packet). The mixture should be thick.

89. Pumpkin Cupcake for Halloween

Ingredients
- products for your favourite cupcake
- products for your favourite cake
- cream pastry cream
- orange pastry
- round cupcake with a hole

Preparation
1. Bake two cupcakes according to your favourite recipe in a round shape with a hole. Allow them to cool in shape and then flip them over to remove them. Cut the bottom of the cupcakes - where they came up when baking - to make them even. Save the clippings.
2. Grease the flat side of one of the cupcakes with your favourite cake cream and blend in with the other.
3. Fill the hole in the middle with the cream-mixed cuts. Spread the pumpkin with the pastry cream outside.
4. Whisk the pastry cream with the mixer until thick and smooth. Paint it with orange pastry paint. Apply the pumpkin - it is already orange.
5. Pour a little of the cream to fill the gap in the middle. Make a "handle" from a celery stalk, or a twig, or whatever you have on hand.

90. Low Carb Nougat Whims

Ingredients
- 210g dark chocolate with a minimum of 70% cocoa solids

- 125 ml (110 g) coconut oil, divided
- 400g coconut milk, only the solid part
- 8 tbsp peanut butter or other nut butter you like
- 1 tbsp (5 g) cocoa powder
- 1 tsp vanilla extract

Preparation
1. Melt half of the chocolate in a water bath or microwave over low heat. Add a quarter of coconut oil and mix well.
2. Pour into a greased mould and coated with baking paper (approximately 13 x 20 inches, if you make 40) and let cool in the refrigerator or freezer.
3. Carefully heat the solid part of the coconut milk (canned) in a different pan. Let it simmer for a few minutes.
4. Add half of the coconut oil, nut butter, cocoa powder, and vanilla while stirring. Make a smooth mixture. If the dough separates, use a hand blender and press several times to make it uniform.
5. Remove from heat and pour over chocolate. Return the pan to the refrigerator or freezer to cool again while the rest of the chocolate melts as in step 1.
6. Add the remaining coconut oil to the chocolate and mix. Spread it in a layer over the cold nougat. Replace in the refrigerator and let stand for at least an hour, preferably longer.
7. Cut into 30-40 small pieces. Store in an airtight container in the refrigerator or freezer. The nougat is best served slightly cold.

91. Raspberry feast meringue with cream diplomat

Ingredients
Preparation of meringue
- 2 egg whites
- 1/2 cup caster sugar
- 1/4 tsp. vanilla extract
- 1/4 cup crumbled barley sugar

Raspberry mousse preparation
- 1 cup frozen raspberries

- 1/4 cup water
- 2 tbsp. Raspberry Jell-O Powder with No Added Sugar
- 1 1/2 cup Cool Whip
- 1 bowl fresh raspberries

Preparation
1. To make the meringue, preheat the oven to 350 o F (175 o C) and line a baking sheet with parchment paper.
2. In a blender or bowl, whisk egg whites until the foam is obtained. Gently add the sugar while whisking until you get firm, shiny picks. Stir in vanilla extract and crumbled barley sugar.
3. Shape the meringues on the coated cookie sheet and place in the preheated oven. Turn off the oven and wait 2 hours. Do not open the oven. Once the meringues are dry, break the meringues into small bites.
4. To make the mousse, put frozen raspberries and water in a small saucepan. Heat until raspberries melt and are tender. Put these raspberries in a blender. Add the Jell-O powder and mix. Once the raspberries have completely cooled, incorporate the Cool Whip.
5. To shape the raspberry, place in balloon glasses for individual portions or in a large cake pan first a layer of raspberry mousse, then a layer of meringue, then fresh raspberries. Repeat the layers. Refrigerate for a few hours before serving.

92. Cheesecake mousse with raspberries

Ingredients
- 1 cup light lemonade filling
- 1 can 8 oz cream cheese at room temperature
- 3/4 cup SPLENDA no-calorie sweetener pellets
- 1 tbsp. at t. of lemon zest
- 1 tbsp. at t. vanilla extract
- 1 cup fresh or frozen raspberries

Preparation
1. Beat the cream cheese until it is sparkling; add 1/2 cup SPLENDA® Granules and mix until melted. Stir in lemon zest and vanilla.

2. Reserve some raspberries for decoration. Crush the rest of the raspberries with a fork and mix them with 1/4 cup SPLENDA pellets until they are melted.
3. Lightly add the lump and cheese filling, and then gently but quickly add crushed raspberries. Share this mousse in 6 ramekins with a spoon and keep in the refrigerator until tasting.
4. Garnish mousses with reserved raspberries and garnish with fresh mint before serving.

93. Almond Meringue Cookies

Ingredients
- 2 egg whites or 4 tbsp. pasteurized egg whites (at room temperature)
- 1 Tbsp. tartar cream
- ½ tsp.
- ½ teaspoon almond extract vanilla extract
- ½ cup white sugar

Preparation
1. Preheat the oven to 300F.
2. Whisk the egg whites with the cream of tartar until the volume has doubled. Add other ingredients and whip until peaks form.
3. Using two teaspoons, drop a spoonful of meringue onto parchment paper with the back of the other spoon.
4. Bake at 300F for about 25 minutes or until the meringues are crisp. Place in an airtight container.

CHAPTER 12: SIDE DISH

94. Pesto Mushrooms

Preparation time: 40 minutes

Ingredients for 6 people
- pepper to taste
- 1 garlic clove
- 200 gr chestnut flour
- 1 glasses of extra virgin olive oil
- 240 gr flour
- 200 gr porcini mushrooms
- 3 tablespoons olive oil
- salt to taste
- 2 thyme sprig
- 4 eggs
- 1 glasses white wine
- 1 bunch of basil
- 1 bunch parsley

Preparation
1. Sifted to the fountain gr. 240 of white flour and gr. 200 of chestnut flour.
2. Add a pinch of salt, break 4 eggs in the center and beat them. Knead the dough until it becomes smooth and homogeneous.
3. Let it rest for 30 minutes, roll out the pastry and cut the noodles. Meanwhile, you cleaned gr. 200 fresh porcini mushrooms, slice them and sauté in a pan with a chopped clove of garlic, 2 sprigs of thyme and 3 tablespoons of oil.
4. Sprinkle the mushrooms with a small glass of white wine, let it evaporate, add salt and pepper and chop them in the mixer.
5. Prepare a pesto with a bunch of parsley, one of basil, 10 peeled almonds, salt, pepper and a small glass of extra virgin olive oil.
6. Mix the chopped herbs with the porcini mushrooms.
7. Cook the tagliatelle and season with the sauce.

95. Lemon Green Beans With Almonds

Preparation time: 20 minutes

Ingredients for 4 people
- Green beans 500 g
- Almonds 120g
- Lemon
- 3 tablespoons Extra virgin olive oil
- 4 tbsp Beetroot leaves
- 150g Salt to taste

Preparation
1. Salad of green beans and almonds
2. Preheat the oven to 180 ° C. Toast the almonds on a baking tray for 5 minutes.
3. Salad of green beans and almonds
4. Add green beans and steam them for about 5 minutes until they are al dente. Emulsify olive oil and lemon juice in a bowl.
5. Salad of green beans and almonds
6. Add a pinch of salt. Put the green beans, almonds and beetroot leaves in a large bowl. Pour the dressing over the salad and mix well. Serve immediately.

96. Sweet and savory brussel sprouts

Ingredients
- a pack of Brussels sprouts
- a shallot
- a tablespoon of brown sugar
- one tablespoon of soy sauce
- 2 tablespoons of apple vinegar
- extra virgin olive oil to taste
- salt and pepper q. b
- a round of balsamic glaze to decorate

Preparation

1. Carefully wash the sprouts, remove the outer leaves, cut them in half and dip them in boiling salted water for ten minutes.
2. Meanwhile, stew a thinly sliced shallot in a pan with a drizzle of extra virgin olive oil.
3. Add the drained sprouts from the water, the spoon of soy sauce and season well for ten minutes. Also, add the apple vinegar and let it evaporate and the sugar making caramelize a few more minutes until completely cooked.
4. Season with salt and pepper and serve with a drizzle of balsamic vinegar glaze.

97. Caramelized sweet potatoes

Ingredients
- 1 kilo of small potatoes, previously peeled and cooked.
- 85 grams of sugar (about 6 tablespoons)
- 75 grams of butter (5 tablespoons approximately)

Preparation
1. We take the potatoes (peeled and boiled) and rinse them in cold water, then dry them and reserve them.
2. Now in a pan over medium heat melt the 6 tablespoons of sugar until it begins to brown.
3. We add the butter to the sugar in the pan, and when we see that the butter stops bubbling we add the potatoes and raise the heat a little.
4. Sauté the potatoes and remove them so that they do not stick or burn. When they are golden we remove them from the fire and serve them.
5. It is not recommended to reheat them, and they are preferably used to accompany meats, either pork or poultry.
6. Enjoy your meal!

98. Vegetable and polenta dish

Ingredients for 2 people
- 125gr polenta

- Vegetables
- 1 eggplant
- 1 mushroom
- 2 celery sticks
- 1 thick branch of broccoli
- 2 small peppers (one red and one green)
- 1/2 medium onion
- 1 cup crushed tomato
- 1/2 glass of water
- 1 teaspoon sweet paprika
- white pepper to taste
- Salt

Preparation
1. First, we wash and cut all the vegetables into strips, slices, and cubes, according to our preference.
2. The bouquet of broccoli is separated into small trees, so as to eat them in one bite.
3. Then, in a large skillet, we put 3 or 4 tablespoons of olive oil. Brown the garlic and onion with a pinch of salt to sweat. We stir for 1 or 2 minutes.
4. When the onion and garlic begin to become tender, add the peppers. We cook 3 or 4 minutes stirring frequently.
5. It is now the turn of broccoli corsages and celery. We add them to the pan and saute together with the rest of the vegetables for 3 or 4 minutes.
6. Finally, we incorporate the eggplant and mushrooms. On this occasion, we are going to lightly resalt the vegetables (especially eggplant and mushrooms) and incorporate the rest of the spices (sweet paprika and white pepper). Stir mixing well for 3 or 4 minutes.
7. Now water all the vegetables with the crushed tomato, and we also add half a glass of water. Remove integrating everything well and cover the pan. Cook over medium heat about 10 minutes, stirring occasionally.
8. Meanwhile, we prepare the polenta. In a pot, we put water, (three times the amount of polenta that we are going to cook) with a teaspoon of salt. When it breaks to boil we slowly add the polenta

in the form of rain, while constantly stirring so that lumps are not made. We cook about 5 minutes stirring constantly until all the water is absorbed. When ready, remove from heat.
9. We incorporate into the pot where we have made the polenta the vegetables with its tomato sauce, mix well and pass everything to the source where we are going to serve the polenta cake with vegetables.
10. Let it cool until the consistency of the polenta hardens and it is easy to cut.

99. Squash fries

<u>Ingredients</u> for 2 people
- 2 medium potatoes
- 1 tbsp olive oil
- 1 salt and pepper to taste

<u>Preparation</u>
1. Cut potatoes into squares
2. Microwave potatoes 1 minute at a time until slightly tender
3. Preheat oil in pan medium heat
4. Add microwaved taters in oil and add salt &pepper
5. Adding chopped onion is optional when heating oil.
6. Cook until desired golden crispiness.

100. Vegetable kebabs

<u>Ingredients</u> for 4 people
- 4 Arabic bread rolls
- half red onion
- iceberg salad to taste
- 600 grams of natural seitan
- spice mix for kebab (cumin, black pepper, sweet paprika, garlic, basil, onion, mustard)
- 1 cucumber
- 1 clove of garlic
- 2 ripe tomatoes

- 250 ml of white soy yogurt without sugar
- apple vinegar to taste
- salt and oil to taste

Preparation
1. We start by cutting the seitan into thin slices (you have to get some "straccetti"), then put them in a pan with some oil, a spoon of the mix of spices for kebabs and about 100 ml of water. Cook and stir, adding flavor until the water is absorbed.
2. In the meantime prepare the necessary for the sandwich. Rinse the salad under running water, dry it with a cloth and cut it into julienne strips.
3. Also, cut the onion into very thin slices and do the same with the tomatoes after having thoroughly washed them. Then peel the cucumber and grate it. Put the obtained pulp in a colander and squeeze it well to remove the excess water.
4. Then prepare the sauce. In a bowl pour the yogurt, oil, salt, a tablespoon of apple vinegar, and the clove of garlic cut in half. Add the cucumber and mix well to flavor all the ingredients.
5. Let the sauce rest in the fridge for about half an hour and remember to remove the garlic before serving.
6. Finally assemble the sandwich. Cut the Arabic bread in half and proceed with the stuffing putting the salad, the tomatoes, the strips of seitan, the onion and finally the yogurt sauce.
7. Enjoy your meal!

CHAPTER 13: Soup and salad

101. Lettuce Wraps with Smoked Trout

Ingredients
For Trout
- 1/2 cup kosher salt
- 2 tablespoons light brown sugar
- 8 trout fillets

For Meyer Lemon Sauce
- 1/4 cup freshly squeezed Meyer lemon juice
- 2 tbsp mayonnaise
- 1 tablespoon full of mustard with grains
- 1 tbsp red wine vinegar
- 2 teaspoons of honey
- 1/2 teaspoon of lemon zest
- Kosher salt and freshly ground black pepper
- 1/2 cup extra virgin olive oil

For Assembly
- 1 packet of butter lettuce, separate leaves
- 1 carrot sliced or grated
- 1 cup fresh parsley

Preparation
For trout
1. Add 4 cups of water, salt, and sugar to a bowl and stir for 1-2 minutes until salt is dissolved. Add the trout fillets and make sure they are covered with saltwater. Close the container and refrigerate for at least 1 hour to 3 hours. Remove trout from saltwater, rinse thoroughly with cold water, and dry.
2. Put the skin on the grilled trout. Put the top plate in the refrigerator and let the trout dry for 21-24 hours or until the skin of the trout is shiny and slightly sticky to the touch. Prepare a sawdust smoker to maintain a temperature of 90 degrees Celsius.

3. Place the trout fillet on the smoker, with the skin down, leaving a gap between them. Adjust the temperature as needed, darken until the trout is cooked, and cook to the desired smoke level for about 20 minutes. Remove the meat from the bones and grate the trout.

Lemon sauce Mayer
4. Mix lemon juice, mayonnaise, mustard, vinegar, honey, and peel, sprinkle salt and pepper in a medium bowl. Add the olive oil slowly and beat until emulsified.

For mounting
5. Put some trout on separate lettuce leaves, sprinkle with a little Mayer lemon sauce, and put carrots and parsley. Wrap the lettuce leaves and help.

Note
If you can't find Meyer's lemon, replace 3 tablespoons of fresh lemon juice and 1 tablespoon of orange juice.

102. Easter salad

Ingredients
- 1 lettuce or lettuce
- 1 parsley connection
- 3 hard-boiled eggs
- 2 tsp mustard
- 3 tbsp oil (olive oil)
- 3 tbsp vinegar
- 1 scallion green onion
- 1 bunch of fresh garlic
- half fried mackerel

Preparation
1. The washed and dried green salad is broken into pieces.
2. The parsley, onion, and garlic are cut very finely.
3. The eggs and fish are cut into thin slices.
4. Beat mustard with olive oil and vinegar.
5. Lettuce, eggs, fish slices and sprinkle with the parsley mix in the salads.

6. Saline.
7. Lastly, pour over the mustard sauce with the mustard sauce.

103. Green salad with grated eggs

Ingredients
- 1 lettuce
- 2 hard-boiled eggs
- 125g yoghurt
- 1 tbsp mustard
- 1 tbsp vinegar
- 1 radish connection
- 50 ml of oil
- parsley
- salt

Preparation
1. The washed and cleaned salad is cut into pieces or broken.
2. Stir in chopped parsley and season with salad dressing with vinegar, salt, oil, and mustard.
3. Stir the mixture and place on plates, pour over the yoghurt.
4. Sprinkle with grated, hard-boiled eggs.
5. Green salad with grated eggs is garnished with red radishes and a sprig of parsley.

104. Green salad with fresh cucumbers

Ingredients
- 1 lettuce or salad
- 2 cucumbers
- 50 ml of oil
- 30 ml of vinegar
- dill
- parsley
- salt

Preparation

1. Salad and cucumbers are well washed.
2. Drain the salad from water and cut it into strips.
3. Peel the cucumbers and cut them into circles.
4. Mix and salt.
5. Drizzle with oil and vinegar.
6. Sprinkle the green cucumber salad with chopped dill or parsley.

105. Green salad with eggs

Ingredients
- 1 salad or lettuce
- 1 radish connection
- 3-4 onions green onions
- 2 hard-boiled eggs
- 3 tbsp oil
- 3 tbsp vinegar
- salt

Preparation
1. Green onions, lettuce, and radishes are cleaned and washed.
2. Cut and place in a bowl.
3. Cut one egg into cubes and add to salad.
4. Stir and cover with a mixture of oil, vinegar, and salt.
5. When serving, the green egg salad is sprinkled with the second egg, grated on a grater.

106. Cold soup with rice

Ingredients
- 500g yoghurt
- 2-3 tbsp rice
- 200 ml of salted water
- 2 hard-boiled eggs
- 1 clove of garlic
- 2 tbsp oil
- salt
- parsley

- cooled water

Preparation
1. For the Cold Rice Soup recipe, the rice is boiled in water.
2. The yolks are ground with oil, garlic, and some salt.
3. The proteins are cut into small pieces.
4. Yolks and proteins are added to the cooled rice.
5. The yoghurt for the Cold Soup with Rice recipe is diluted with chilled water.
6. Pour into prepared mixture.
7. When serving, cold rice soup is sprinkled with finely chopped parsley.

107. Cucumber tar with yolks

Ingredients
- 2 cucumbers
- 300g yoghurt
- 2 eggs
- 1 clove of garlic
- 1 tbsp oil
- 1 tsp vinegar
- 60 ml of water
- dill
- salt

Preparation
1. For the "Cucumber with yolks" recipe, the cucumbers are washed, peeled, and cut into small cubes.
2. The eggs are cooked firmly and, when cooled, peeled.
3. The yolks are separated and grazed.
4. Add yoghurt to the paste yolks successively, stirring with a wire to form a creamy mixture, water, crushed garlic, some chopped dill, salt, vinegar, some of the oil.
5. Mix well and add finely chopped cucumbers.
6. The cucumber-yolk recipe mixture is stirred again and refrigerated.

7. When serving, the yolk of cucumbers with yolks is watered with the remaining oil and sprinkled with dill.

108. Winter chickpea soup

Ingredients
- chickpeas - 1 jar
- tomatoes - 1 pcs.
- onions - 1 head
- celery - 2/3 of the stem
- carrots - 2 pcs.
- parsley - 5 stems
- garlic - 1 clove
- cow butter - 3 tbsp.

Spices
- rosemary, savoury, paprika, salt, turmeric, curry

Preparation
1. Clean and wash chickpeas, onions, and carrots, then drain them well and put the oil in a preheated pot.
2. When it is melted, we add the vegetables and simmer to take in the butter.
3. During this time, peeled tomatoes, celery, parsley, and garlic in a chopper and cut them until a paste-like mixture is obtained.
4. After chopping them, add them to the other vegetables in a saucepan.
5. Season and mix well so that the ingredients do not start to fry.
6. Pour hot water into the pan and cook the vegetable cream until all ingredients are ready.
7. Once everything is cooked well enough, we remove the pan from the hob and fry everything well.
8. To make it more nutritious and saturated with chickpeas, you may want to add some cooking cream.

CHAPTER 14: Meat dish

109. Veal rolls with stuffing and mushroom sauce

Ingredients
Stuffing
- mushrooms - 200g or mushrooms or a mix of both
- white wine - 50 ml
- yellow cheese - 4 slices Emmental or other
- onion - 1/2 head
- Indian curry - 1/2 tsp qualitatively
- salt - to taste
- black pepper - to taste

About the border
- nutmeg - 2 - 3 tongs
- salt
- pepper
- parsley - 2 tbsp
- onion - 1/2 head

Mushroom sauce
- mushrooms - 15g dried
- mushrooms - 300 g
- oil - 2 tbsp.
- flour - 2 tbsp.
- pepper
- salt to taste
- curry - 1/2 tsp quality Indian
- white wine - 180 ml
- water - 100 ml

Preparation
1. Cut the mushrooms into strips and the onion into small pieces. Stew them in a pan with a little cow butter. Add the wine to glaze

the mushrooms and onions. Cook until wine is evaporated. Allow the mixture to cool. Using lightly oiled hands, shape the border by first flattening it into schnitzels. Place one slice of yellow cheese and the mushroom stuffing.
2. You close the rolls in the form of a salt roll, the numbers for this quantity being 4. Arrange the veal rolls in a saucepan and put in an oven at the bottom of which you poured 50 ml of wine and baked at 180 degrees for about 20-25 minutes or until you notice that a tangy tan begins to form.
3. While baking the rolls, prepare the mushroom sauce. Cut the fresh mushrooms into strips.
4. Break the dried mushrooms into pieces and mix them with water in a small bowl. Allow the mushrooms to rehydrate for 15 minutes. Drain the soaked mushrooms while preserving the liquid. If you don't have dried mushrooms, skip this step!
5. In a small saucepan, melt the butter over medium-low heat. Add the fresh mushrooms and chopped onions and fry them. After about five minutes, add the flour, salt, pepper, and curry and mix well.
6. Add the white wine, the soaked mushrooms, and their liquid and cook for 5 to 7 minutes, until the sauce is thick enough and the bubbles come out.
7. When the veal rolls are baked, add the baking sauce to the aromatic mushroom sauce.
8. Serve the delicious veal rolls with stuffing and mushroom sauce cut into mushroom sauce.

110. Medfune

Ingredients
- lamb - about 500 g
- eggplants - 2 large
- green peppers - 3
- onions - 2 heads of chromids
- garlic - 1 crushed clove
- sugar - 2 tsp
- salt - 2 - 3 tsp

- coriander - 1/2 tsp dried
- olive oil - 3 - 4 tbsp.
- bags - 1 tsp
- cinnamon - 1/2 tsp

Preparation
1. The eggplants are washed and cut in lengths. They are salted and allowed to drain from the mustard, then rinsed with salt, placed in a pan, sprinkled with olive oil and baked in the oven until ready.
2. The lamb is cleaned of veins and zippers, cut into small pieces as much as a bite, mixed with the onion and cinnamon sliced in slices, and left to cool in the marinade for one hour.
3. The olive oil is heated in a pan, the cloves of garlic are released, and the meat is added, stirring constantly.
4. When the meat remains fat, add the second onion and peppers, salt, sugar, and spices, cut into slices, mix, slam with a lid and cook until ready.
5. The roasted eggplant halves are cut in the middle, placed from the meat stuffing, and the stuffed eggplants returned to the pan back in the oven until slightly red.
6. The stuffed Medfune eggplants are served with a sprinkle of olive oil.

111. Pork stew with prunes

Ingredients
- pork - 500 g
- onion - 1 pc.
- black pepper - 1 tbsp
- tomato puree - 2 tbsp
- salt
- black pepper - 7 - 8 pcs. grains
- bay leaf - 1 pcs.
- beer - 1/2 can
- parsley - fresh connection
- rum - 50 ml
- dried plums - 150 g

Preparation
1. Soak the prunes in the rum and leave them there.
2. Wash and cut the meat into bites.
3. Put some fat in the pan and add the meat inside. Wait for the water to boil and remain greasy.
4. Put onions, which you previously cut into retail. Fry for a few minutes.
5. Add the red pepper and tomato paste, and after a few minutes, the beer.
6. Wait for the alcohol to boil and pour some water.
7. Put the spices on, reduce the stove, and let the pork stew simmer for half an hour under the lid.
8. Squeeze the plums from the rum and add them to the pan.
9. Close and allow the pork with plums to simmer for half an hour or until meat is cooked.
10. Serve pork stew with dried plums warm sprinkled with fresh parsley.

112. Classic meatballs with tomato sauce

Ingredients
- mince - 250 g
- Onion - 1/2 pc.
- parsley - 1/2 connection
- bread - 1 branch
- salt
- pepper
- Eggs - 1 pcs.
- flour - for oval
- FOR THE SAUCE
- Onion - 1 pc.
- Carrots - 1 pc.
- celery - a stalk
- garlic - clove
- salt
- red pepper - 1 tbsp
- sugar - 1 tbsp

- tomato puree - 100 g
- tomatoes - 500g fresh

Preparation
1. Put the border in a large bowl. Cut onion and parsley into retail. Put them on edge.
2. Add salt, pepper, egg, and soaked bread in water - drained. Knead the border.
3. Make small balls. Roll the meatballs in flour and flatten them lightly.
4. Put some fat in the pan and fry them gently on both sides. Take out and set aside.
5. Put the onions, carrots, and celery in the same fat that you previously cut into retail. Stew until soft.
6. Add the tomatoes cut into small pieces, tomato paste, and red pepper. Pour some water.
7. Put salt, sugar, and pepper.
8. Press the garlic using a garlic press. Stir, reduce the heat and allow the tomato sauce to boil for one hour.
9. Remove from the hotplate. Gently mix the sauce with the blender. Return to the hotplate.
10. Put the meatballs inside and cook for another 10-15 minutes.
11. Remove the meatballs with tomato sauce and sprinkle with fresh parsley.

113. Stuffed chicken legs

Ingredients

For the legs
- chicken legs - 4 pcs. (deboned)
- ham - 80g boiled or sausage, bacon, and more.
- mozzarella - 80 g
- pickles - 30 g
- salt

Spices
- truffle oil - to taste or extra virgin olive oil
- cow butter - 50 g

- blueberries - 50 g
- white wine - 100 ml
- hot water - 100 ml
- flour - 30g for oval legs

About the kawerma
- onions - 4 heads
- red peppers - 2 pcs.
- duck leg - 200g or mushrooms, mushrooms
- tomatoes - 100g (or 1 tablespoon salt, diluted with 100 ml water)

Preparation
1. First, you debone your chicken legs (or buy ready-made deboned chicken legs).
2. Marinate the legs with salt and pepper, optional spices/coriander, black pepper, chilli pepper, cumin, turmeric or rosemary and salvia / and truffle oil for about 60 minutes.
3. Cut the ham, mozzarella and pickles, and whatever you like. Add about three to 4 blueberries to the mixture for each leg. Fill the legs.
4. Wrap them well with a kitchen thread (or toothpick) to prevent the cheese from leaking during cooking. Finally, grease the legs with extra virgin olive oil and roll in the flour.
5. Seal stuffed legs on all sides in heated cow butter. Pour the wine and the same amount of water.
6. Stew in a pressure cooker or Multicooker for about 20 minutes.
7. Cut onions and red peppers. Heat the oil in a frying pan and simmer for 10 minutes. Add the mushrooms and simmer for another five minutes. Then add the stewed vegetables to the chicken legs and cook the broth for another 15 minutes.
8. Enjoy your fillet with stuffed chicken legs.

114. Crochet with lamb brain

Ingredients
- Lamb brain - 2 pcs. / or other animals in an amount of about 1 h

- bread - 1 dry slice, soaked in fresh milk and drained
- Eggs - 1 pcs.
- onions - 1 head of chromed
- Cow butter - 2 tbsp.
- salt - 1 tsp.
- white pepper - 2 - 3 tongs
- breadcrumbs
- oil - for frying

Preparation
1. The lambs' brains are cleaned and soaked in cold water for at least one hour, then dried, removed with a zipper, and rubbed into a bowl through a coarse strainer or a small saucepan.
2. Grind the onion or grind very well and stew in the oil until softened, mixed with salt and pepper.
3. It is cooled, and, along with the broken bread, the egg and egg are added to the shredded brains. Everything is mixed well, and 1-2 tablespoons are added if needed. breadcrumbs.
4. Allow the stretch film to cool for half an hour, then form croquettes.
5. They are rolled into breadcrumbs and fried in the oil of a medium-hot plate.
6. Finished lamb brain croquettes are left to drain from grease on kitchen paper.

115. Pumpkin and apple soup

Ingredients
- 450 grams (1 lb.) pumpkin
- 1 Granny Smith apple cored, and quartered
- One medium onion cut
- Two cloves garlic
- One tablespoon of olive oil
- salt
- ¼ teaspoon of cayenne more to taste
- 300 ml (1¼ cup) of vegetable stock
- freshly ground black pepper to add taste

Garnish
- pomegranate arils
- some pumpkin seeds
- fresh parsley finely chopped

Preparation
1. Preheat the oven about 200 degrees C (or 392 degrees F). Line a large baking sheet with a parchment paper.
2. Cut the pumpkin half lengthways and scoop out seeds.
3. Slice each pumpkin half in half to make quarters and place, cut-side up, on a baking tray, along with the onions.
4. Drizzle with olive oil and then sprinkle some salt.
5. Bake for about 20 minutes, then add the garlic and apple, flip the pumpkin cut side down and then roast for another for 20 minutes, or until the flesh is soft.
6. Use a spoon to scoop out the flesh of the pumpkin and transfer to a high-speed blender with the apple, onion, garlic (remove the skins), cayenne, and vegetable stock.
7. Blend on high for almost 2 minutes, or until silky smooth.
8. If too thick, add vegetable stock to thin it out and blend over. Taste and adjust the seasonings.
9. Serve, ladle soup into a bowl, and with pomegranate arils, pumpkin seeds, fresh parsley and freshly ground black pepper.
10. Then serve.
11. Refrigerate leftovers inside an airtight container for 4 days.

116. Reds salad on bacon and balsamic vinaigrette

Ingredients
- Balsamic vinaigrette:
- ¼ cup olive oil
- Three tablespoons balsamic vinegar
- ½ teaspoon finely chopped garlic
- ¾ Dijon mustard spoon
- ¾ honey bee teaspoon
- Salt and pepper to taste

- Salad with red grapes, bacon, and walnut:
- 3 cups mixed lettuce (escarole, French, ball, Italian)
- ½ cup red grapes, in halves
- Two slices of bacon, golden brown
- 8-10 praline or natural walnuts
- Two tablespoons blue cheese, Roquefort or blue cheese

Preparation
1. Balsamic vinegar vinaigrette:
2. Mix all ingredients in a jar, cup or dish and mix well until everything is well incorporated.
3. Add season to taste.
4. Salad with red grapes:
5. Cook the bacon until well browned and cut into medium pieces.
6. Mix the lettuce with half of the balsamic vinaigrette.
7. Place on a plate.
8. Add the red grapes in halves, the bacon in pieces, the blue cheese, and the nuts.
9. Serve with the remaining vinaigrette.

117. Arugula, lettuce and strawberry salad

Ingredients
- ¼ red onion, thinly sliced
- 4 cups of arugula leaves
- 250g tapered strawberries
- 90g goat cheese crumbled
- 1 to 2 cases of balsamic vinegar
- 2 to 3 cases of olive oil
- The salt according to your taste

Preparation
1. Dip the onions in cold, lightly salted water to remove the bitter side.
2. Mix the balsamic vinegar, olive oil and salt in a tight container and shake to the rhythm of the salsa.
3. Drain the onions and mix with the arugula leaves and the vinaigrette.

4. Top with crumbled cheese, sliced strawberries, and spicy pecans.
5. Mix at the table and serve immediately.

118. Curry tuna salad

Ingredients
- 400g natural tuna one beautiful romaine 100g raisins two medium pippin apples one lemon juice one teaspoon curry 1 cup mayonnaise

Preparation
1. Open the can of tuna. Drain and divide into large pieces.
2. Wash and dry the salad leaves thoroughly. Peel apples before cutting into thin slices sprinkle the lemon juice to prevent them from turning black.
3. Dressing the tuna salad with curry:
4. In a salad bowl, arrange the salad leaves, the pieces of tuna, the raisins and the slices of apple to mix everything.
5. Add the curry to the mayonnaise and stir well.
6. Mix the mayonnaise with the salad just before serving.

119. Roasted carrots and cashew salad on lemon vinaigrette

Ingredients for 2 people
- 4 beautiful carrots
- One wrist of cashew nuts
- One wrist of parsley or coriander
- One tablespoon soup grape dry
- For seasoning:
- One lemon
- One tablespoon of tahini
- Two tablespoons of olive oil
- One tablespoon of hazelnut oil

Preparation

1. Peel the carrots and grate them. Put them on a serving plate. Mince the parsley and add to the carrots. Add the raisins on top.
2. Heat 1 tablespoon of vegetable oil in a skillet over high heat and sauté the cashews. Stir frequently, so they do not burn. When they turn a beautiful golden color, place them on paper towels and salt them. Let it cool before adding them to the carrots.
3. Prepare the seasoning: squeeze the lemon and place the juice in a bowl. Add the tablespoon tahini and mix well with a fork to fully dilute the sesame puree. Add two tablespoons of olive oil including a tablespoon of hazelnut oil. Mix the sauce well to incorporate the oils.

120. Baby spinach, chicken and carrot salad with red wine dressing

Ingredients
- Carrots: 2
- Red onions: 3
- Spinach sprouts: 80 g
- Olive oil: 3 tbsp. soup
- Lemon juice: 0.5 tbsp. coffee
- Juice of 1/2 orange
- Agave syrup: 1 tbsp. coffee

Preparation
1. Peel the carrots and onions. Cut the carrots into slices using a thrifty knife and sliced onions.
2. Wash the spinach sprouts, and then drain them. Mix in a medium bowl with the carrots and onions.
3. Mix the agave syrup with the olive oil and the orange and lemon juice. Pour over the salad and mix before serving. Enjoy it immediately.

CONCLUSION

This diet, which is largely inspired by the Mediterranean diet, certainly helps reduce the risk of contracting a cardiovascular disease or a chronic inflammatory disease. It is easy to follow and is balanced as no food group is totally put aside; it is more about consumption frequencies to respect.

Although the anti-inflammatory diet is generally good for health, it is especially suitable for treating some health problems. For example, the anti-inflammatory diet reduces the risk of heart disease, keeps existing heart problems under control, reduces blood pressure and triglycerides in the blood (natural fats formed by the combination of fatty acids and glycerol) and soothes hard rheumatic joints. This diet aims to increase physical and mental health by recommending healthy, fat, fiber-rich fruits and vegetables, abundant water, and a limited amount of animal protein (excluding fish), providing a constant source of energy and reducing the risk of age-related diseases.

Made in the USA
Coppell, TX
08 January 2020